COVIDSLAYERS

How We Can Win!

And

What Really Went Wrong?

A Physician Leader's Experiences From The Frontlines

Rajesh Mohan, MD, MBA, FACC, FSCAI

COVIDSLAYERS

Copyright©2020 Rajesh Mohan

All rights reserved

The views expressed in this book are solely of Dr. Rajesh Mohan's and do not represent those of North Atlantic Medical Associates, P.C, Lakewood, New Jersey, RWJBarnabas Health, New Jersey, Monmouth Medical Center, Long Branch, New Jersey, Monmouth Medical Center, Southern Campus, New Jersey, Community Medical Center, Toms River, New Jersey, Jersey Shore University Medical Center, Neptune, New Jersey, or any other associated and unassociated entity, entities, group or individual both in the past or present with which Dr. Mohan may have been, or deemed to be, associated with. This book was undertaken as an outside activity separate from Dr. Rajesh Mohan's official duties associated with any and all of the above entities and organizations. Any statement, phrase, discussion related to any medicine, disease or treatment in this book are opinions and not medical advice. No interpretation of this book should be taken as medical advice. The author does not assume any responsibility for any omissions or inaccuracies. Any resemblance or attribution to any person or group of people, living or dead, unless stated by name is purely coincidental, unintentional or in the public domain either within an organization or in the public sphere. The characters and events portrayed in this book, unless referenced by name, are fictitious. Any similarity to real persons, living or dead, is coincidental and not intended by the author.

No part of this book may be reproduced, or stored in a retrieval system, or transmitted in any form or by any means, electronic, mechanical, photocopying, recording, or otherwise, without express written permission of the author.

ISBN-9798564305662

Library of Congress Control Number: 2018675309

Printed in the United States of America

COVIDSLAYERS

Table of Contents

Acknowledgements 1
About the Author 2
Introduction 3
Chapter One 8
The Sirens Were Blaring 8
Chapter Two 18
The Real (Not the Fake) Panic 18
Chapter Three 26
When the Cavalry Is Delayed 26
Do It Yourself – Do Not Wait 26
Chapter Four 32
Guidelines for Convenience 32
and 32
CDC's Fall from Grace 32
Chapter Five 52
Science and Logic Became Dispensable 52
Chapter Six 59
Misplaced Priorities 59
Healthcare Is About Patients First, Stupid! 59
Chapter Seven 76
Bigotry and Humanity—In a Pandemic 76

Chapter Eight	84
The Dogma of Bureaucracy	84
Chapter Nine	94
The Inhumane Visitors Policy	94
Chapter Ten	102
Strategies to Combat COVID-19	102
Chapter Eleven	123
Let us Fix It – It is about time!	123
Chapter Twelve	140
The Warriors, The Martyrs - All Heroes	140
Epilogue	145
Bibliography	152

Acknowledgements

My parents, Janak and Dr. Aryma N. Srivastava, for their teachings and my upbringing which have made me the person I am. I have been taught to be strong, resilient and speak up in the defense of right and fight against wrong. I have been taught by them to never take anything for granted, always work hard, and leave nothing to chance. If we all had followed my parents' teachings and advice, I believe, we would not have had thousands of preventable deaths of our fellow Americans due to the COVID-19 pandemic.

My wife, Nandini, for her unconditional love and support. She has always been a pillar of strength. She encouraged me throughout the process of writing this book, going through multiple drafts, and helping me keep my focus despite negative forces emanating from different directions.

My sons, Yuvraj and Vishvajit, for keeping me grounded and inspiring me to continue to put forward my best possible efforts to improve lives.

My patients, who have given me the reason and confidence to touch more lives and endeavor to make a positive difference in the lives of as many people as I possibly can.

My physicians, nurses, and other healthcare friends and colleagues, who have the common goal of a better healthcare system so that we can provide timely and efficient patient care and help improve lives and livelihoods of our fellow Americans.

About the Author

Dr. Rajesh Mohan is a quadruple board certified, fellowship trained interventional cardiologist. As the Chief Medical Officer of a hospital located in one of the early epicenters of the COVID-19 pandemic in the U.S., and a practicing physician, he led from the front, managing the initial surge of the COVID-19 pandemic.

Anticipating the severity of the disease, he successfully planned and implemented multiple key strategic initiatives in the fight to beat back the onslaught. Actively seeing and treating COVID-19 patients on the frontlines, he was one of the first proponents of early rather than late treatment of such patients. Working with community leaders and his team of physicians, he led outreaches to the local community in the middle of the initial surge, educating the public to seek early medical attention.

Dr. Mohan has held multiple leadership positions including serving as the Chair of Medicine and has taught medical students, residents, and cardiology fellows, serving also as an Assistant Professor of Clinical Medicine for several years. He has been recognized for leading, innovating, and implementing strategies to improve patient care, and aligning key stakeholders for institutional success. Dr. Mohan has been the recipient of multiple leadership and academic awards. Dr. Mohan is board certified in Internal Medicine, Cardiology, Nuclear Cardiology, and Interventional Cardiology, and has an MBA.

Introduction

My mother always says, "when you honestly give your hundred percent in the service of the good to overcome evil, you will always come out victorious because the blessings and strength of God and the people will be with you."

It appears that mothers of all frontline healthcare personnel must have said the same to them growing up. This book is a tribute to the valor and strength, the grit and sacrifice, the compassion and resilience, and the persistent lionhearted heroism against all odds of healthcare personnel. Frontline healthcare personnel have been the only source of inspiration during this pandemic. In this once-in-a-100-year pandemic, it is the profound acts of courage of physicians, nurses, nurses' aides, respiratory therapists, environmental services and other frontline healthcare personnel, who have fought (and are still fighting) valiantly that have stemmed the rising tide of preventable deaths of our fellow Americans.

This is a story of the war against the Coronavirus disease 2019 (COVID-19) pandemic from the frontlines and from war rooms. It is a unique perspective from a practicing physician and a clinical administrator and those of his colleagues at various hospitals and medical practices who treated COVID-19 patients on the frontlines, planned combat strategies in the battlefield as well as orchestrated strategies in the war room and then implemented them on the frontlines, while fighting alongside a team of exceptionally gifted fearless warriors.

With no cure and no vaccine, physicians have dug deep into their banks of knowledge, training, experience, and critical thinking. It is their

COVIDSLAYERS

propensity for innovative thinking and the mission to improve lives – the reason why they went to medical school – that has helped them conceive management strategies to treat COVID-19 patients. From the seemingly common and over-the-counter supplements and vitamins to major surgeries such as double-lung transplant and heart-lung transplant have been used as treatments in attempts to help COVID-19 patients recover and save lives.

With rationed N95 masks and personal protective equipment (PPE), nurses and nurses' aides have spent hours taking care of COVID-19 patients at the bedside, sweating within their gowns and masks which they used multiple times. Only the most compassionate of humans, and certainly not the faint of heart, would endure such extreme conditions with smiles on their faces lest the patients become despondent. They served as surrogates for family members and held the hands of dying patients, with a stoicism that belied the volcano of pain, anguish and tears that flowed only after the passing of life that they had been tending to.

Respiratory therapists, intensivists and anesthesiologists braved the virus infested air and fumes of breathing treatments, while intubating COVID-19 patients during their courageous efforts to help gasping patients get some air.

Environmental services personnel worked in fear, with a blend of sweat and tears behind their masks, trying to clean and disinfect isolation rooms which may have been saturated with the virus during the stay of a COVID-19 patient who died and had just been taken down to the morgue.

Healthcare personnel who are on the frontlines – from the registration desk, the emergency department, through the hospital and down to the morgue, who are battling this pandemic have unlimited courage, grit, and compassionate hearts.

This book is also about the failures of our healthcare system in combating this pandemic. The COVID-19 pandemic laid bare our unhealthy healthcare system, which was found wanting when Americans needed it the most. The failures were systemic.

Without a real understanding of the failures and making corrections, we will be at risk of repeating them again. The book may ruffle some feathers and may appear to be critical of public officials, health officials, administrators, policymakers and politicians; and it may very well do so because they owned it – for better or for worse.

Healthcare leaders or healthcare generals (in the war against the pandemic), who were supposed to lead this war against the pandemic, have been humbled by it.

The leaders of our healthcare system failed to effectively mount an offensive against the virus. It is immaterial whether these leaders realized the gravity of the pandemic or not, whether they assessed the threat adequately or not, or whether they planned adequately or not. When the war became a reality, did they act responsibly and with competence? Who else would or should have, if not them? Who failed the American people? Who failed the frontline warriors?

It was not just the politicians. Healthcare administrators and public health officials share the responsibility and the blame equally, if not more.

If we want to progress in healthcare so that we can take care of each other and our fellow Americans, then the first step should be to own up to the failures and the reality that has been laid bare by the COVID-19 pandemic. It has made it obvious that our healthcare administration is not as good as we think.

Not surprisingly, it has shown that the clinical care provided to patients in the U.S. as most of us have always known, is better than many give it credit for. Sadly, the pandemic has also made it evident that the high quality, top-notch clinical care provided to patients in the U.S. has been, over the years and during this pandemic, compromised by healthcare administrators and politicians.

After more than 240,000 Americans dead in just about 9 months, there must be a reckoning with the truth. We still have a long way to go before we vanquish this virus. Currently, the virus is winning the war and human lives and livelihoods are being lost daily.

The way we rise from the quagmire of our unhealthy healthcare system is by owning up and manning up to our shortcomings, facing them and correcting them. It cannot be and must not be back to business as usual. The

COVIDSLAYERS

current healthcare leaders/generals should own up, take responsibility, and become part of the solution. Our inability to remediate failures caused by the insecurities of administrators and politicians should not be the reason to continue down a proven failed path. We do need some administrators in healthcare, maybe not as many. The worthy ones will remain essential elements of healthcare. The paper-pushers will fall by the wayside. The active physician and clinical administrative leaders should not shy away from taking the lead. In fact, they must take the lead.

Very importantly and pertinently, this book explains smart strategies to contain COVID-19 and ultimately vanquish this pandemic. Included are various mitigation tactics as well as containment strategies like the Directly Observed Self-isolation and Contact Tracing (DOS-CT) and eDOS-CT, which should not be overbearing to the public.

Urgent containment of the COVID-19 pandemic is essential until a cure or a vaccine is easily available to all Americans.

We must find strategies that are smart and not extreme. Extreme strategies such as a total lockdown should be reserved only for desperate and extreme situations where everything else has failed and there are no other options. Extreme tactics or strategies do not get the buy-in from the populace and therefore they generally would not work, especially in a free and democratic society as ours.

We must stop the deaths and mayhem caused by COVID-19. If we do not, then until a cure or a vaccine becomes readily available, there will be continued death and destruction of American lives. Even if a cure or a vaccine is eventually available to all Americans, currently and in the year ahead, smart strategies, if implemented, are the only paths to prevail over this pandemic and avoid more deaths, loss of jobs, livelihoods – extensive, and in some cases irreparable economic costs to individuals and our country.

If we all unite, then together we all will vanquish this pandemic and come out of this stronger and better and will rise as COVIDSLAYERS!

Dr. Rajesh Mohan

COVIDSLAYERS

Chapter One

The Sirens Were Blaring

Friday the 13th, March 2020.

COVID-19 (COVID, Coronavirus disease 2019) was approaching town.

As a physician and the Chief Medical Officer (CMO) of a hospital, blaring sirens do not typically faze me. Practicing as an interventional cardiologist for about two decades, I had become adept at routinely managing unexpected and exigent situations any time of the day or night. To be woken up at 2:00 AM to immediately transform one's thoughts and actions to function at a sustained rapid pace calibrated to meet varying patient needs, including making life impacting decisions had become second nature, and was not the least bit disconcerting.

I do not consider this to be a unique attribute that I have been selectively imbued with; rather, one that finds its genesis in the nascent stages of medical school and is cultivated through the years. These are skills developed, begrudgingly at times, working what seem like inhumanely long hours and placing patients and medicine over friends and family that contributed to my remaining calm and reflective as the tempest around me began to brew.

In the clinical and administrative role of a CMO, in addition to seeing patients as a practicing cardiologist over almost two decades, the unflappability that had become embedded over the years as a cardiologist would help me in managing situations ranging from the mundane to the threatening, including bomb threats.

Could one individual, one hospital, one community, one state, or even one country, be able to successfully manage the tsunami of a lethal pandemic that was enveloping the entire world? – I wondered. It was patently obvious that a coordinated and concerted effort and planning was required with the buy-in of ALL stakeholders, ranging from the warriors on the frontlines to the politicians, public officials, health officials, administrators, and policymakers in board rooms. It would only be then that there would be a realization among the general public regarding the gravity of the threat to not only their personal lives and the lives of their loved ones but also to their livelihoods and the "routine" lifestyle that most had become accustomed to.

Knowledge and education, truth and honesty, transparency and accountability provide the most strength in any war where an efficient and successful outcome leading to victory is the goal. It would only be due to the power derived from this strength that the general populace would come together organically to vanquish this pandemic. It was obvious that the warriors on the frontline – the boots on the ground, were acutely aware of this. If others were going to take the looming crisis seriously or not, only time would tell. I had a sinking feeling that it was not going to be the case.

The proof is always in the pudding. With over 240,000 Americans dead in only about 9 months and counting, the pudding did not come out well.

It was going to be a survival of the fittest – I surmised.

March 1, 2020 was when New York (NY) state had its first confirmed case of COVID-19. The World Health Organization (WHO) had announced

COVIDSLAYERS

on March 11, 2020 that the COVID-19 outbreak was officially a pandemic. On March 13, 2020, with 421 cases, New York State had the highest number of confirmed COVID-19 cases in the United States. From the time that NY state had its first COVID confirmed case, it took only 13 days for it to achieve the dubious honor of No. 1 in the US in terms of having the most COVID-19 cases. New York City had started contemplating closing public schools.

The President of the United States declared a national state of emergency on March 13, 2020.

March 4, 2020 - the first positive COVID-19 patient was announced in the state of New Jersey (NJ). In the early days and up to the first weeks of March, in the state of New Jersey, tests were still mostly being conducted by the New Jersey Department of Health (NJDOH) which would then go to the Centers for Disease Control and Prevention (CDC) for confirmation. Unfortunately, even with the obvious warning signs at the time, top health administrators in NJ were providing unfounded pollyannaish advice to the political leadership and the public proclaiming that most New Jersey residents were at very low risk of contracting the virus.

Really! Only people with shallow or no knowledge about an infectious disease pandemic with a combination of arrogance or naivete would have come to that baseless conclusion – I thought.

In a stark reminder of the ignorance and callousness of administrators and policymakers, even when testing at private laboratories was limited in New Jersey and as late as in the middle of March, so-called directives were being sent to physicians, stating that they "must" obtain specimens for COVID-19 tests "in their office" and to "use their normal courier service or send the patient with specimen and prescription to a Quest or LabCorp lab".

This, for obvious reasons, did not make much sense!

It was apparent to physicians that to collect nasopharyngeal swabs for COVID-19, adequate Personal Protective Equipment (PPE) with a minimum of N95 masks, face shields, gowns and gloves are required. It was common knowledge that PPE was (and continues to be) intentionally or unintentionally, in limited or restricted supply. N95 masks, if available, were being sold at premium price – they still are. The same was true for other required PPE. In addition, asking possible COVID-19 patients to go to physician offices would have risked other patients and the office staff to potential exposure to COVID-19. Not all physician offices had staff that were trained or equipped to obtain adequate samples for COVID-19 tests. COVID-19 tests at that time, and long thereafter, had a turnaround time of 4–7 days for results to be obtained. Most importantly and the obvious fact was, that if major hospitals and medical institutions were having a shortage of tests, how in the world were individual doctors' offices (who are not only much smaller entities with limited resources when compared to hospitals) expected to obtain COVID-19 test kits.

It was obvious that these so-called directives were coming from influential policymakers and administrators who had limited knowledge of both our healthcare system as well as the management of a pandemic.

The COVID-19 pandemic had arrived in New Jersey. One could feel the beginning of the pandemic in New Jersey with a sense that the tsunami had already reached its shores.

Governor Phil Murphy declared a state of emergency in New Jersey on March 9, 2020. The first fatality due to COVID-19 in the state of NJ occurred on March 10, 2020. In the state of NJ, by March 13, 2020, the total number of COVID-19 cases had reached 50, with one death. New Jersey hospitals had already begun seeing an increasing number of admissions of suspected COVID-19 patients.

It was only a matter of time before the situation would get worse.

On March 13, 2020, I received more phone calls than usual. Not surprising for a Friday – I call them "Friday specials." But this Friday seemed different – most calls were about COVID-19. The anxiety levels were at a scale that was unlike those that I had sensed or experienced before.

My cell phone rang – a friend and colleague, who is also a critical care physician sounded concerned, anxious, and maybe even scared.

Dr. Kumar said, "I think I have COVID-19."

COVIDSLAYERS

Dr. Kumar went on to describe his symptoms, which were very suggestive of COVID-19. He also stated that he had an exposure to a possible COVID-19 patient at a hospital. I asked him to go to the emergency room so he could be immediately looked after.

Dr. Kumar went to the emergency room (ER), was evaluated, tested, and then decided to go home to self-isolate while he waited for the results.

Dr. Kumar went home knowing in his mind that he had COVID-19 but hoping that he did not.

Wishing Dr. Kumar the best, I arranged a rapid COVID-19 test with a turnaround time of about 24 hours for him, as he was essential personnel in the fight against COVID-19. Rapid was about 24 hours to results at the time!

When I later spoke to Dr. Kumar, he had already started himself on high dose Vitamin C, Zinc and Vitamin D3. In addition, he had bought a pulse oximeter and a thermometer. He stated – "I cannot believe I had such a hard time finding acetaminophen (Tylenol) and the vitamins." Americans were emptying stores of such items and more. Panic and panic buying had already begun.

While I had a sense of this all day long, the conversation with Dr. Kumar served as both confirmation as well as a harbinger of things to come. The blaring sirens that never seemed to faze me before, were no longer background white noise that years of training had made me accustomed to; rather, their frequency, both in numbers and decibels, were becoming increasingly difficult to ignore.

Healthcare personnel were apprehensive and were bracing for the worst. Physicians across hospitals were being approached by nurses and hospital staff for advice and reassurance. My physician friends and colleagues experienced interactions with nurses and hospital staff who inquired if it was even safe to go to work or interact with COVID-19 patients. Physician leaders were being asked how they would be testing and treating patients if we did not have enough tests and no known treatments. There were questions and frustration expressed regarding COVID-19 test results, which at the time took 4-7 days.

Healthcare personnel as well as the public were receiving conflicting and frequently changing information from administrators and healthcare agencies. Not surprisingly, nurses and frontline healthcare personnel turned to get answers from clinical physician leaders in hospitals who they worked with closely, and as a result trusted their knowledge and expertise more than they trusted administrators and state and federal government healthcare agencies. Many answers were being sought for questions such as those listed below, from trusted clinical physician leaders by frontline healthcare warriors in many hospitals.

What do we do? Is it safe to come to work? Should we stay home?

What is the availability of N95 masks? When should we wear it and when should we not?

There is no treatment. What are we going to do with all the patients?

How do we know if anyone has COVID-19 if we do not get the test results in time?

How will we treat them if we are waiting for 5 days for test results?

When confronted with similar questions myself, I would, in addition to trying to answer their questions based upon Centers for Disease Control and Prevention (CDC) and the Department of Health (DOH) guidelines, express my solidarity and empathy with the staff. I also tried to bolster their confidence by stating – "stay strong, we will find a way and together we will come out of this stronger and better." This would become my mantra for the days and months since.

Clinical physician leaders across hospitals were responding and leading efforts to improve transparency and diminish anxiety levels among healthcare personnel. There were meetings including townhalls that were being scheduled in hospitals in addition to the command centers that were being set up, where questions from healthcare personnel would be addressed. There was a heightened sense of awareness with reality being established among physician leaders that COVID-19 was on the shores of NJ and was knocking on doors of hospitals in NJ. Physician leaders sensed the anxiety and high stress levels among their fellow healthcare personnel and concluded that, at a minimum, they were owed the reassurance and confidence that they were not in this battle alone.

Most questions that healthcare personnel had in these meetings at various hospitals were related to PPE and COVID-19 tests or the lack thereof, and the resultant challenges that could potentially negatively impact patient care and the safety of healthcare personnel. Questions such as:

Were there enough tests? How soon can we get the results of the test? What do we do while we are waiting for the test? Who can order the test? On what patients are the tests to be ordered?

What about visitors? Were family members allowed? What were the entry points?

Should the patient wear a mask in the room?

Was on-site outpatient blood draw going to be stopped?

Are we doing terminal extubations in COVID-19 patients?

What are the guidelines for COVID-19 testing?

The schools were going to be closing – what about childcare?

Were we going to allow hospital volunteers?

Were we going to cancel outpatient services?

Were we going to do elective surgeries?

When patients are being transported to and from the hospital, were we going to screen emergency medical personnel, and if so, how?

What are we doing to test asymptomatic COVID-19 patients?

All these questions and more were being asked, even before the first COVID-19 patients were being admitted in many hospitals in the state of NJ – and rightly so!

I have always believed that the frontline staff and what I like to call them – boots on the ground – always have a greater and better appreciation of reality than many administrators in boardrooms. That is why I have also believed that the best administrators are those who not only have regular interactions with the boots on the ground, but also spend a portion of their time *as* boots on the ground.

It was widely believed that many clinical physician leaders and nurse leaders were physically present and interacting with other healthcare personnel at all hours of the day and night in various hospitals. It was also becoming increasingly apparent that the only way to get a true sense of any hospital staff's capabilities and comfort level of managing COVID-19 patients (from their perspective) was to be among them, listen to them and to answer their questions honestly and to the best of one's ability. A direct one-on-one conversation would also help keep the messaging consistent with the boots on the ground. Since the situation was not only unprecedented but exceptionally consequential for both the hospital staff as well as the patients who would walk through the hospital doors, it would be good for the morale of the hospital staff if they experienced transparency from their clinical leaders who they trusted more than any other healthcare administrator or agency.

Communication, transparency, and accountability were the only things that would help give them the confidence to do what they do best – which is to take care of patients.

All hospitals and healthcare personnel, after all, were about to stand face-to-face with possibly the worst pandemic in almost 100 years. This was not the time to lead from behind or from an office. It never is!

The general sense among clinical physician leaders across hospitals was that, as healthcare personnel in hospitals in New York and New Jersey were becoming more and more involved in direct and open and transparent conversations, rising anxiety levels were tempered and diffused to some extent, although most still persisted due to the distrust of public health officials, government agencies, politicians and administrators.

However, what would shine through about every physician, nurse, respiratory therapist, nurse's aide, phlebotomist, environmental services and other healthcare personnel was the overpowering force – of fortitude and steel, that each one of the boots on the ground had. There was no one who wanted to beat a hasty retreat. In fact, the questions, and clarifications, for the most part, pertained to how best to manage the crisis, how best to protect each other, and how not to carry the infection home to families. No one was running for the hills.

Healthcare warriors were readying up to take the fight to the virus, save as many patients as they could, protect each other from the virus and protect their families by not taking the virus home – battles on different fronts, all at the same time!

It was war – against a barely known and an invisible enemy.

Reaching home around midnight that Friday, after a quick shower and dinner, I lay in bed recollecting the events of the past about eighteen hours. That day, I could not have been prouder to serve shoulder to shoulder with the staff that I had seen grow and mature over the past three plus years.

Dr. Rajesh Mohan

Chapter Two

The Real (Not the Fake) Panic

Next day, Saturday, March 14, 2020, I woke up early. I had to get back to the hospital!

Although I was not "on-call," there was no way that I could not go.

I did during the day, what I did the day before – a repeat of what I did on Friday - interacted, listened, and answered questions. Together with senior nurse leaders, I went to each floor and unit throughout the hospital. We met with multiple physicians, nursing staff and hospital staff, listening and communicating with them. There was a need to allay the fears constantly and repeatedly. The concerns and the anxieties had to be acknowledged, respected, and addressed on an ongoing basis. It could not have been a one and done. This was going to be an ongoing crisis, at least for the near future.

Ordering some pizza may have helped! Providing pizza/lunch to staff helped, as it was one less thing that they needed to worry about. Although, in retrospect, I do not think many even had an appetite. It was very evident that the questions and anxieties would keep surfacing no matter how many times or how often they were addressed. In fact, about nine months after the initial onslaught of COVID in the U.S., the questions and anxieties still persist not only in hospitals but among the general public throughout the country – in some regions more than others.

By the weekend, clinical physician leaders, physicians, nurses, and other healthcare personnel were feeling the need to establish command centers in various hospitals. It could not have waited until Monday! There was no dearth of volunteers to staff the command centers.

Later that evening, I received a message from the laboratory, which was given to me as per Dr. Kumar's instructions. Dr. Kumar was positive for COVID-19!

I called Dr. Kumar, informing him of his results and enquiring from him about his well-being. His first reaction was not about himself but the fact that he was disappointed that he would not be able to join the fight against the pandemic for at least two weeks, especially because he had high fever and shortness of breath on exertion. I advised him that he should first take care of himself and that he must not hesitate in coming to the hospital if needed. He agreed. I also requested him to not worry about the hospital and instead to focus on taking care of himself and getting better soon.

Hospitals were being asked to prepare and increase their critical care beds and, with that, their critical care nurses and physician staff. Many hospitals were increasing their critical care beds by almost 50 to 100 percent or more.

Plans are only good if they are approved, so that they can then be executed.

Clinical hospital leaders in many hospitals knew what it would take from a physician and nursing staffing perspective if the number of critical care beds were going to be increased to high numbers as expected so as to be able to take care of the unprecedented numbers of COVID-19 patients that were being expected. The clinical leaders across hospitals were ready with plans and ready to go. But the execution of all these plans is dependent upon the financial administrators. Finance folks usually insist on observing a demonstrated need over a sustained period of time before they approve additional healthcare personnel, while the working physicians and nurses on staff continue to be squeezed to their last drop. This model of staffing need assessment may be an appropriate model for assessment and decision making in non-healthcare sectors, but this approach is detrimental on so many levels when human lives are at stake.

In many hospitals, there is usually one hospitalist physician at night from 7:00 PM to 7:00 AM who would sometimes be responsible for taking care of about 50 plus patients on a usual night. In some places this lone hospitalist physician also takes care of critical care patients and admits patients from the ER. With COVID-19 approaching, many clinical leaders had come to the conclusion that it would not only be unfair and unsafe to patients and the lone physician, but also exasperatingly thoughtless to expect that one physician to take care of such sick and complicated patients throughout the night all by himself or herself. Even under "normal" circumstances, expecting one physician to take care of about 50 patients, including critical care patients, in addition to admitting patients from the emergency room, is not normal and should not be normalized.

In healthcare, physician and nurse staffing should be trimmed only when waste and expenses in all other departments and areas of a hospital and other entities have been minimized to the maximum. Finance based attrition, if at all, should only be applied to the two pillars of healthcare - physicians and nurses, which have direct patient care consequences, as a last resort. There is more than enough waste and inefficiency in healthcare administration that must be eradicated before any financial cuts are contemplated in areas that provide direct clinical care to patients. Healthcare entities are in existence primarily for taking clinical care of patients – everything else must be secondary.

I had a strong group of hospitalists (internal medicine doctors) and private practice physicians who spanned the spectrum. They included physicians who were internists, intensivists, cardiologists, infectious disease specialists, hematologists, anesthesiologists, nephrologists, some surgeons, and a few radiologists. Although a small group, these physicians proved that they belonged to the segment of healthcare personnel who had the highest ethical and moral standards. They truly showed that the cliched statement that being a physician is a calling is actually a reality. This group of physicians was the backbone and the power of the physician response to COVID-19 at our hospital. They were later joined by intensivists from across the country, who came in as reinforcements to bolster our fight in our war against the pandemic.

Driving home around midnight on Saturday, March 14, 2020, although I was apprehensive, I was also cautiously optimistic about the preparation for our hospital that we had put together locally, over the past few weeks. At our hospital, we had developed plans to combat the pandemic. We had the capability to follow through with some items in those plans. However, some other items in our plans were dependent on others and outside help. Many of the items that we were dependent upon for outside help were critical. These included PPE, testing capabilities, ramping up critical care physician / intensivist staffing, increased number of critical care nurses and nurse staffing for the medical floors, more respiratory therapists, conversion of critical care and medical floor COVID cohort rooms to negative pressure rooms, more availability of dialysis machines and personnel to operate them, to mention some.

We just had to convert our plans into action without further delay, at least the ones that we could on our own and were not dependent on outside help for – it was time!

My main concern remained that other than the hospital staff and boots on the ground, many others, for the most part, had until that point not taken the pandemic as seriously as they needed to. There was still a lot of bureaucratic dragging of feet. This was not only true about many in the political sphere, many healthcare administrators, and policymakers but, also among the general public, many in healthcare related businesses as well as non-healthcare businesses. They continued to be to a large extent pollyannaish even until then!

COVIDSLAYERS

Some consequential policies were finally being formulated and sent for implementation that Friday, March 13, 2020, while some were probably going to be mulled over the weekend for implementation on Monday, March 16, 2020, by the so-called policymakers. Meanwhile, doctors, nurses, and individual hospitals had no choice but to stop waiting for such policies and guidance and instead come up with their own. Visitor policy, suspension of volunteer services, isolation criteria, PPE usage, screening of visitors and patients, testing for COVID-19 both by NJDOH as well as by private laboratories – policies, processes and guidance for all these and more should have been formulated and sent out at least 2-4 weeks in advance.

Remember, the first case in New Jersey was on March 4, 2020. All this was not that difficult to fathom and should have not only been anticipated, but completed and ready to deliver, if not already delivered. The preparedness for all the stated items, policies and guidance should have been organized in advance and made available to be deployed at a moment's notice. The inevitable onslaught of the pandemic was a foregone conclusion. It was not a matter of if, but when.

Since January 2020, many physicians had raised concerns and asked that COVID-19 be taken seriously. This was true not just of physicians who were on the frontlines and boots on the ground – locally and across the country but also some clinical physician leaders. In the beginning, physicians across the country were asking, and then imploring, that there be a process for easy testing. This should have been aligned with self-isolation coupled with contact tracing. These requests from physicians across the country were dismissed by politicians and administrators and public health officials with explanations that included that "it would create panic." Some healthcare and hospital administrators responded to such requests of starting the process for COVID-19 testing stating that they did not agree with frontline physicians and clinical physician leaders.

I have always believed that transparency and honesty, especially while facing a crisis, is always better than the fear of the unknown.

How would testing and knowing if one has a disease or not create panic when we know that people could be potentially exposed sooner or later, anyway? – I asked myself. With this warped logic, women should not have a mammogram to know if they may or may not have breast cancer or people should not have a colonoscopy to know if they may or may not have colon cancer or someone should not have a test for Human immunodeficiency virus (HIV) if they want to know if they may have been infected after a suspected exposure.

Instead, public and health officials treated the American people in a condescending manner. Americans can handle the truth. Americans understand responsibility. Americans should have been treated as adults by politicians, public officials, health officials and administrators.

We had already started admitting patients who were suspected of COVID-19. We just did not know for sure if they were confirmed positive for COVID-19 or not. The turnaround time for test results was about 4-7 days. This was due to the lack of availability of COVID-19 tests and the absence of a preplanned efficient operation to process the tests in a timely manner. This was directly a result of the incompetence of, and lack of anticipation by, many non-believer public officials, health officials, administrators, and policymakers!

I wished that the public officials, health officials, policymakers and administrators were half as anxious and scared as the hospital staff!

But wait! Many of these administrators, policymakers and public officials did not have to venture out of their offices or homes! Many were getting ready to move into the safety and comfort of their homes, with their families, to "work from home." They did not have to be on the frontlines or come face to face with patients who were infected by the virus and their families or have the direct responsibility to take care of sick COVID-19 patients. They did not have to struggle against all odds to try to make these patients better and then send them home to their loved ones who would be apprehensively waiting for them all that time, not having been allowed to visit them in the hospital by these very public officials, administrators and policymakers. Why would they be anxious and scared – they just had to push paper?!

COVIDSLAYERS

After taking a quick shower and dinner after midnight that Saturday, I lay in bed wondering, like I am certain many of my physician colleagues were, if administrators would have any regrets about not trying to get ahead of the virus a month in advance. Protocols and procedures which were now being prepared and implemented on the fly and in a chaotic manner could have had multiple dry runs by now!

I wondered if those administrators across hospitals and healthcare were now spending sleepless nights reconsidering their decisions to NOT promote testing or publicly acknowledging the crisis, which would have evoked the appropriate and timely public response and handling of the pandemic.

Were they up rethinking the applicability of "what you don't know can't hurt you," in the medical field?

Nah! I said – they must be sound asleep.

Dr. Rajesh Mohan

COVIDSLAYERS

Chapter Three

When the Cavalry Is Delayed

Do It Yourself – Do Not Wait

Sunday, March 15th, 2020.

Command centers across hospitals developed dashboards that would keep track of all suspected COVID patients, pending COVID tests, confirmed COVID patients, daily COVID and non-COVID patient census, daily COVID test results – negative and positive, COVID cohort bed availability, intensive care unit (ICU) bed census, ventilators – in-use and available, nurse staffing, respiratory therapist staffing, number of N95 masks, tally of surgical masks, gloves, gowns, and face shields and their availability, morgue availability, and so on.

As patients were already being admitted with suspected COVID-19 and test results were still pending, regular guidance to nursing staff, physicians and other hospital staff became essential. This was even more consequential as policies, guidelines, recommendations, and directives were coming from different agencies at varying speeds. Some lagged behind another and some were repetitive but were released in a different time frame with the potential of causing or adding to the confusion. Making sure that there was adequate provision of masks and PPE for nursing staff, physicians and other direct patient care providing healthcare personnel became important. Command centers in hospitals became not only a central location for daily tally of all available PPE but also a coordinating center for allocation of PPE to all departments as well as nursing units.

The process was dragged out at various hospitals, partly due to the inertia inherent to the bureaucratic structure of hospitals and their procurement processes, in general. There was also a tug of war between clinical healthcare personnel and non-clinical administrators in hospitals who controlled the procurement process for N95 masks and PPE. It did not help that CDC, the premier national and international organization that was supposed to be an expert in managing pandemics, kept changing their guidelines and recommendations regarding masks and PPE.

To many physicians and nurses, science and established best practices were not being followed in these guidelines. Instead of making sure that there was adequate manufacturing and supply, as well as an efficient procurement process for masks and PPE, science was being bent to justify new guidelines. These new guidelines gave cover to supply chain personnel and administrators at various hospitals to hide behind. It made it easier for them to express their helplessness and justify their incompetence in procuring an adequate supply of masks and PPE, and instead use the CDC guidelines as an excuse to ration PPE to frontline healthcare personnel and boots on the ground. It was disingenuous, at the very least!

COVIDSLAYERS

The tsunami had started engulfing New Jersey while it was devouring New York. Patients suspected of COVID-19 had started being admitted to hospitals in New Jersey. Many of these patients suspected of COVID-19 were placed in COVID cohort rooms, in isolation, at various hospitals. Healthcare personnel who would go into these COVID rooms were provided with and asked to wear masks and PPE. They were asked and expected to discard the masks and PPE when leaving these isolation rooms. This was based upon established science and best practices.

However, outside the units and in the hospital hallways, many hospitals did not allow masks due to the concern and fear of carrying the infection from an infected patient's room to other areas. In addition, how would one know or police anyone who continued to wear the same mask coming out of a COVID or any other isolation room. This scenario became even more likely with masks and PPE being rationed. Prior to COVID, no one thought twice about discarding masks, gloves, and gowns at the time of leaving an isolation room – they were discarded. No one in their right mind would continue to wear the same masks, gloves and gowns coming out of any isolation room. They were disposable and for one time use only. There were plenty and kept outside each patient's room. It was different now. Now they were not readily available, especially outside each patient's room. They were now being hoarded by hospitals, and many were under lock and key and then rationed.

Throughout the day, in news stories and among physicians, nurses and other frontline healthcare personnel in conversations and on social media, there continued to be more questions and concerns regarding masks and PPE more than any other topic. COVID-19 testing was a close second.

Frontline warriors – nurses, environmental services and other healthcare personnel across hospitals were becoming increasingly scared and apprehensive and felt like they were sheep being sent for slaughter. Some even wanted to quit and go home – to fight another day – with appropriate body armor (PPE). The reason they stayed behind was because of their strong hearts and their faith in each other and the physicians and clinical leaders who fought by their side.

Dr. Rajesh Mohan

Many physicians and clinical administrative leaders at hospitals realized that they had an extraordinary responsibility toward the hospital staff, the medical staff and nursing staff, while making sure that patients were being taken care of in the best possible way. This sense of responsibility was different, as many had not experienced such a personal threat to life while trying to save lives, which they routinely did before. Never before this once-in-a-100-years pandemic were healthcare personnel themselves so overwhelmingly at a significant mortal risk, while trying to take care of patients and save lives.

Many of my physician and physician leader friends and colleagues at various hospitals made a resolution to themselves that they would do everything in their power to make sure that all hospital staff, until the crisis was over, shortage or no shortage, were adequately protected and have access to appropriate PPE. Many physicians and medical staff members donated money and tried to make it easier for staff to access N95 masks. It appeared that physicians and some healthcare personnel were able to procure N95 masks faster and easier than many hospitals despite price gouging.

Politicians could have easily mandated increased production under the Defense Production Act, which would have prevented price gouging. Businesses could have still made money if they had increased production and not seemingly indulged in wartime profiteering, even if they had no altruistic leanings, no sense of service or any societal obligations. Healthcare personnel were ready to and paid more for PPE and N95 masks due to the prevalent price gouging as they knew that their lives, the lives of their fellow colleagues and the lives of their family members were more valuable while they valiantly fought battles to save others, including some with contrarian values.

Healthcare warriors at various hospitals wished that administrators, politicians, hospitals and healthcare agencies who had deeper pockets, more resources and power, would have at least a fraction of the moral values that presumably reside at the core of any individual or entity in or linked with healthcare.

The time to wait for the cavalry to come was long past gone!

COVIDSLAYERS

Physician administrative leaders in many hospitals devised plans to assure procurement of N95 masks and other PPE, work closely with supply chain personnel and keep a close eye on disbursement of all masks and PPE. In addition, they increased their one-on-one interactions with frontline healthcare personnel taking direct care of COVID-19 patients and encouraged them to call them directly if anyone refused to give them appropriate PPE.

And they did!

On more than one occasion almost daily, over the first few days, calls from nurses on the floor expressing their difficulty in obtaining N95 masks or some other PPE would be received by clinical leaders who then took matters in their own hands to ensure the real-time delivery of required PPE. The initial frequent incidents exhibiting nurse's frustration and anguish waiting outside the room of a COVID-19 patient while N95 masks and appropriate PPE were being delivered so that he or she could then safely go into a patient's room to take care of the patient were common in many hospitals.

Physicians, for the most part, (in addition to donating) were able to search the market and buy N95 masks for themselves (they should not have had to, the hospitals should have made sure that they had enough) and depended less on hospital resources or the lack thereof.

Supply and distribution of N95 masks and other PPE to hospital staff continued to be sluggish and rationed across many hospitals.

Dr. Rajesh Mohan

Chapter Four

Guidelines for Convenience

and

CDC's Fall from Grace

Monday, March,16 2020, people in New Jersey knew that the COVID-19 pandemic tsunami had started making an impact.

In the state of New Jersey, hospitals and hospital staff were readying themselves to face the tsunami. Most apprehensions and questions from the boots on the ground in hospitals continued to relate to masks, PPE and COVID tests. On the other hand, the media, administrators, policymakers, and the politicians had ventilators on their mind – most conversations were about ventilators. Yes, we did need more ventilators. But it was masks, PPE and COVID-19 tests that were the need of the hour, and then ventilators!

However, it was all about ventilators and ventilators all the time. Maybe ventilators were a more sensational or sexier topic!

In hospitals across the state, COVID Command centers was getting calls about N95 masks, PPE, COVID-19 tests from hospital staff, nurses, and physicians. These command centers were fielding anything, and everything related to COVID. There continued to be frequent changes in policies and guidance from CDC, DOH, the state, as well as from many hospital systems.

It was frustrating and infuriating that there was no planning of any significance for the manufacturing and procurement of N95 masks, other masks, gloves, gowns and for that matter *any* PPE, at *any* level. It was incomprehensible that in an *infectious disease* pandemic, basic requirement of PPE for healthcare personnel was not thought worthy of any coherent thought process and planning. As a result, PPE which, when not routinely required in the past and was readily available then in substantial quantities, became a scarcity when needed the most. Limited availability and subsequent rationing of masks and PPE was akin to sending troops into battle without any body armor!

CDC threw away their own recommendations for best practices about infection prevention and PPE and were changing their "guidelines" on a frequent basis so as to be able to justify the limited availability of PPE and subsequent rationing even where they were needed the most – in hospitals. This continued through the week. Physicians, nurses, and healthcare personnel were and still are finding it difficult to understand, rationalize and most importantly have belief in some of the so-called new and changing guidelines – many of them contrary to established science and best practices. Many such guidelines and directives appeared to be made merely for the convenience of administrators, so that they were able to justify the lack of procurement and availability of masks and other PPE. These so-called guidelines appeared to be welcomed by the administrators who often use(d) them for the purpose of hiding their incompetence and lack of financial alacrity.

N95 masks and other PPE are essential during patient care to not only prevent exposure to healthcare personnel from COVID-19 and other infections, but they are also supposed to be discarded after every patient interaction so that there is no transmission of COVID-19 and other infections from one patient to another and to other personnel. The situation was worsened due to delay in results of COVID-19 tests which resulted in an increased usage of PPE as staff could not presume that patients whose tests were pending were COVID-19 negative and therefore had to use PPE with any patient interaction until the results were back.

Until the pandemic, to prevent cross-contamination and transmission of infection as a cause for healthcare associated infections (HAI) from patients who may be carrying an infection, healthcare personnel were always advised to discard masks and PPE when they exited a patient's room. Now, with a highly contagious virus – COVID-19 – this would be even more of a concern. However, with the rationing and limited availability of masks, gowns and other PPE, there was concern that if masks and PPE are limited, then what would prevent nurses, respiratory therapists, doctors, environmental services personnel, nurses' aides, and others from walking around the hospital with the same masks and PPE, potentially contaminated with COVID-19 or any other infectious agent.

All these masks, gowns and other PPE were made to be *disposable* and for *one-time use only* – as per the manufacturers and CDC guidelines and best practices until recently – prior to the pandemic!

Chaos reigned during the initial days! The unnecessary chaos reeked of a bigger problem – apparently there were a significant number of people lacking in competence who were in positions of power, policy and decision making. The worst-case possibility was – if these policymakers and administrators knowingly (or unknowingly – if one wants to give them the benefit of incompetence instead of willing negligence) did not want to grasp the gravity of this pandemic and its consequences (which had become increasingly apparent), and therefore, underplayed the approaching catastrophe and kept their heads in the sand. Any one of these possibilities in any level of variation was not only tragic for the public, but also for the boots on the ground. This was in many eyes, management malpractice and gross negligence.

Dr. Rajesh Mohan

Communications were being sent out in many hospitals with recommendations for masks, PPE, and COVID-19 testing that were based upon guidelines and recommendations being sent from CDC, DOH and hospital systems. Medical and hospital staff were asked to refrain from wearing masks, gloves, and gowns outside patient rooms as per the guidelines, unless they had a documented flu exemption. In addition, masks and PPE were supposed to be discarded upon leaving rooms of patients who had or were suspected of having COVID. Due to the gravity of the situation – with a highly contagious virus potentially in our midst and to prevent its spread, in addition to the spread of other infectious agents, among patients and hospital staff – many hospitals were trying to enforce these recommendations and guidelines – some more than others. There was little room for error or indiscriminate practice in the midst of a deadly pandemic.

With the confusion and chaos that was prevalent, sooner or later there would be some variation in practice. Some nurses and physicians, especially in the ER would insist on wearing masks outside patient rooms. Some would even insist to do the same in the medical units and the ICUs. Many in the hospital, nursing and medical staff were apprehensive about others wearing masks, gloves and gowns outside patient rooms and contaminating keyboards, workstations, doorknobs, computers, mouse and so on. There was also concern about possibly spreading infections by individuals who would not discard masks upon coming out of patient isolation rooms. At the same time, they were also concerned about getting infected themselves if they did not wear masks, gloves, and gowns outside patient rooms, especially if some decided to wear them.

On March 17, 2020, there was a study published in the New England Journal of Medicine and reported by The New York Times that suggested that COVID-19 could live for three days on surfaces such as plastic and steel, and for twenty-four hours on cardboard.

There was also an increasing number of studies and reports that the COVID-19 virus was also airborne, although according to the New York Times, on March 17, 2020, "the World Health Organization (WHO) had until then referred to the virus as not airborne." However, it was abundantly clear to doctors that airborne infection and spread of the virus was a distinct possibility which was now being reiterated by expert scientists with the recommendation that "surgical masks are probably insufficient."

To many physicians and some healthcare personnel, it was becoming increasingly apparent that community spread of COVID-19 might already be present. If not, it was only a matter of days – a couple of days. Mask wearing within the hospital in the hallways and outside patient rooms was becoming increasingly common, with physicians leading the way. The hope was that those masks worn outside of patient rooms would not be the same that were worn inside patient rooms, especially isolation and rooms with COVID-19 patients and that they would be discarded appropriately.

Early in the week, hospitals in NJ had still not progressed to universal masking. However, as the week advanced, there was an intense and increased demand by physicians and nurses to do so. Based on science, most medical professionals across hospitals were convinced that universal masking to combat community spread of COVID-19 should be implemented, but guidelines and recommendations from the CDC, DOH and health organizations said otherwise. No physician leader wanted their hospital staff, medical staff, and nursing staff to get unnecessarily exposed to the potentially deadly virus if all that was needed was wearing a mask.

CDC's new guidelines had the potential to thwart the capabilities of the boots on the ground who were fighting the fight of a century. It was apparent that there was not much of any real educated or rational thought process involved. These guidelines were only going to serve as impediments and roadblocks to the good fight.

Despite knowing the science and possessing knowledge about COVID-19, the CDC continued to give cover to policymakers and administrators for their lack of planning and incompetence.

Under the cover of stupefying CDC guidelines, the American Hospital Association stated that "surgical masks are an adequate substitute when a supply of N95 respirators is not available, citing the Centers for Disease Control and Prevention's recent decision to relax its own guidelines."

No! A surgical mask is not "adequate," as it is "not protective against inhalation of a pathogen from the cloud," as per researcher Lydia

Bourouiba, an associate professor directing the Fluid Dynamics Transmission Laboratory at Massachusetts Institute of Technology (MIT), an expert in characterizing and modeling infectious disease dynamics and transmission at various scales.

A Change.org petition signed by more than 450,000 healthcare providers in the middle of March 2020 which later increased to more than a million signatures urged for the production of more critical supplies – PPE and N95 masks. In the petition they also wrote that "recommendations.... should not be made based on what's available; availability should be based on what is necessary." The petition indicated that as a result of the recommendations from the CDC which were in response to supply chain challenges, "many hospitals have taken the CDC recommendations to mean that facemasks are the preferred PPE, rather than a less desired (and potentially less safe) alternative. They have thus rationed respirators...." The petition stated that a "Harvard study in China that suggested health care workers were at a 20% increase risk of severe infection compared to the general public. The risk decreased once the Chinese implemented full gear: protective suit, medical goggle, face shield, and N95 mask and gloves – following this change there were no further reports of infected health care workers."

AHA's lobbying alert also stated that surgical masks were *sufficient protection*. AHA was also pushing the narrative that N95 masks were not required during routine interactions between healthcare personnel and COVID-19 patients. The Executive Director of the National Nurses Union, the largest nurses' union, correctly responded – "It is unfortunate that the American Hospital Association is encouraging its member hospitals to adopt minimum rather than optimum standards to protect patients and the doctors, nurses and other staff who care for them. In the face of an exploding pandemic, running backward is the worst approach the health care industry, and the CDC, should take."

If the tussle over N95 masks was not enough, even surgical masks became scarce and precious commodities. The president of the American Health Care Association and National Center for Assisted Living stated that "The CDC guidance came out telling people not to use N95 masks. That helps with the supply of N95s, but it puts a greater burden on the supply of surgical masks."

It would have been absurdly amusing if it were not ludicrous and tragic. So, what were the nurses and doctors supposed to use to protect themselves and their family members from this highly contagious and potentially lethal virus?!

The American Medical Association (AMA), the so-called major professional association for doctors, wrote to Vice-President Mike Pence emphasizing the need for more N95 respirators and surgical masks, in a feeble attempt to keep itself relevant. The AMA and many other major medical organizations were mostly absent and rendered themselves inconsequential in the biggest story of their lifetimes.

Many COVID-19 patients who were admitted to hospitals would deteriorate rapidly. As a result, they would require rapid intubation to be placed on a ventilator. The anesthesiologists or intensivists who would intubate these patients along with the respiratory therapists were at high risk of exposure and risk of infection during this procedure. As a result, not only N95 masks were essential but PAPR (Powered Air Purifying Respirator) devices are considered to be preferable "in situations in which a live airborne virus is being handled," as when aerosolized virus is being spewed in air while a COVID-19 patients airway is being manipulated during intubation. A PAPR is known to provide "a higher assigned protection factor (APF) than N95 FFRs (filtering facepiece respirators)." Therefore, as per the CDC, "a PAPR can be used for protection during healthcare procedures in which HCP (healthcare practitioners) are exposed to greater risks of aerosolized pathogens causing acute respiratory infections." It also goes on to say that "PAPRs provide increased protection and decrease the likelihood of infection transmission to the wearer as compared to FFRs and half face reusable elastomeric respirators."

Anesthesiologists, intensivists, and respiratory therapists in hospitals were imploring for PAPRs. These PAPRs could be used multiple times as long as appropriate cleaning protocols were followed – unlike the N95 masks which were made for one time use only. PAPRs were in demand and apparently ordered by hospitals but were not delivered weeks into the raging battle that frontline healthcare personnel were gloriously fighting.

Administrators were being asked – "Is anyone using PAPRs for….intubation?"

The response was – "Just so everyone knows they cost $1300 each. We cannot offer these unless that is the absolute recommendation from the CDC which…..believe at this point it isn't."

No wonder, the PAPRs were not being delivered! The floundering CDC could not make up its mind about many, if not all, recommendations, and guidelines about COVID-19. It was for the most part either fumbling or flip-flopping. Apparently, the CDC had no gumption to propose an "absolute recommendation" about anything related to COVID-19 in the foreseeable future.

Many healthcare agencies and hospitals claim to be unabashed proponents of "the culture of safety" – of patient safety and employee safety. Many of these healthcare agencies are not in the trenches and do not directly take care of patients, including during this pandemic. They are comprised of bureaucrats who went into hiding and were afraid to step into hospitals even to observe if "patient safety" and "employee safety" was being practiced in real-time. They would undoubtedly be back after the fact to review papers to either sermonize or give token citations or small fines. Many ex-clinicians as well as non-healthcare personnel, have made alternate careers in healthcare as administrators, promoting themselves as messiahs of safety. The patient safety industry was a $1.9 billion dollar industry in 2019 and is "projected to reach USD 2.2 billion by 2024."

However, for these messiahs of safety, essential armor for the purpose of employee safety such as N95 masks, PAPRs, other PPE and COVID-19 tests required for timely patient care did not seem to be important enough.

COVIDSLAYERS

N95 Mask

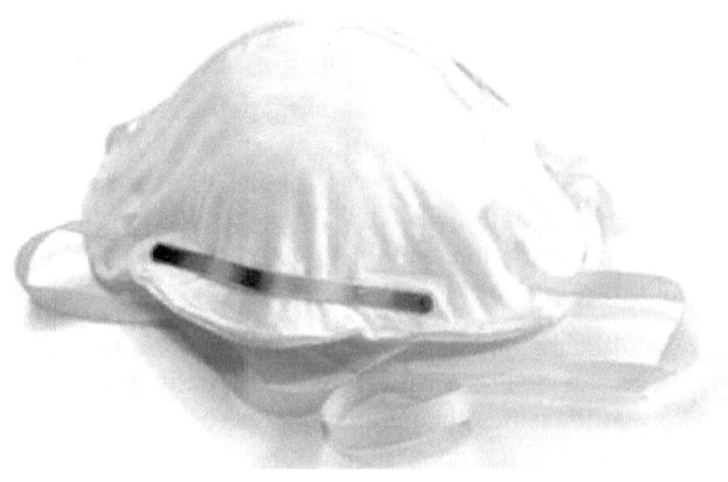

Picture Credit: U.S. Food and Drug Administration
https://www.fda.gov/files/n95_respirator.jpg

Dr. Rajesh Mohan

<u>Surgical Mask</u>

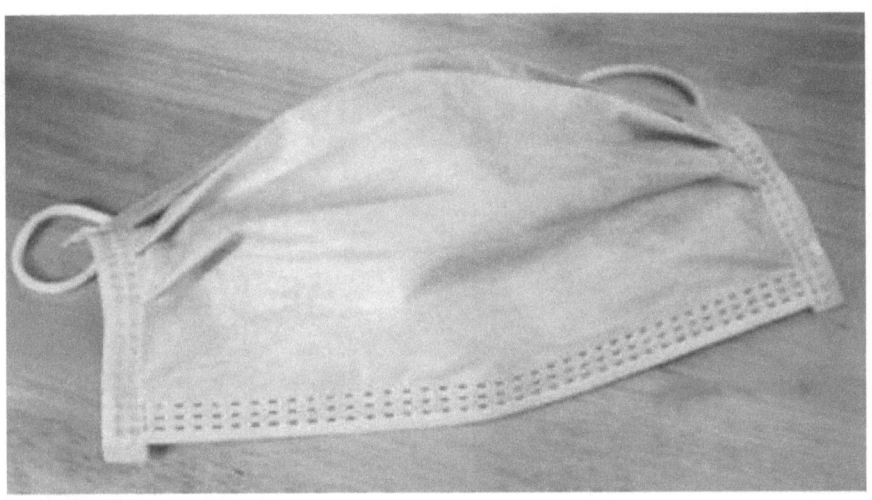

Picture Credit: U.S. Food and Drug Administration
https://www.fda.gov/files/surgical_mask_0.jpg

COVIDSLAYERS

Air-Purifying Respirators

What are Air-Purifying Respirators?

Air-purifying respirators (APRs) work by removing gases, vapors, aerosols (droplets and solid particles), or a combination of contaminants from the air through the use of filters, cartridges, or canisters. These respirators do not supply oxygen and therefore cannot be used in an atmosphere that is oxygen-deficient or immediately dangerous to life or health. The appropriate respirator for a particular situation will depend on the environmental contaminant(s).

Filtering Facepiece Respirator (FFR)

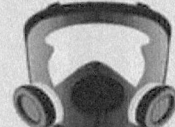

- Disposable
- Covers the nose and mouth
- Filters out particles such as dust, mist, and fumes
- Select from N, R, P series and 95, 99, 100 efficiency level
- Does NOT provide protection against gases and vapors
- Fit testing required

Elastomeric Half Facepiece Respirator

- Reusable facepiece and replaceable cartridges or filters
- Can be used to protect against gases, vapors, or particles, if equipped with the appropriate cartridge or filter
- Covers the nose and mouth
- Fit testing required

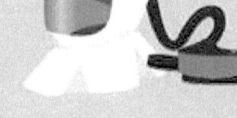

Elastomeric Full Facepiece Respirator

- Reusable facepiece and replaceable canisters, cartridges, or filters
- Can be used to protect against gases, vapors, or particles, if equipped with the appropriate cartridge, canister, or filter
- Provides eye protection
- More effective face seal than FFRs or elastomeric half-facepiece respirators
- Fit testing required

Powered Air-Purifying Respirator (PAPR)

- Reusable components and replaceable filters or cartridges
- Can be used to protect against gases, vapors, or particles, if equipped with the appropriate cartridge, canister, or filter
- Battery-powered with blower that pulls air through attached filters or cartridges
- Provides eye protection
- Low breathing resistance
- Loose-fitting PAPR does NOT require fit testing and can be used with facial hair
- Tight-fitting PAPR requires fit testing

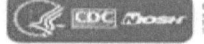
Centers for Disease Control and Prevention
National Institute for Occupational Safety and Health

Picture Credit: Centers for Disease Control and Prevention

https://www.cdc.gov/coronavirus/2019-ncov/images/hcp/N95-infographic-What-Are-APR-508.png?noicon

Their stark callousness broke through the facade and exposed their lack of concern for employee safety as well as patient safety. However, the disingenuous but sophisticated lip service to the culture of safety remained ubiquitous lest anyone see through the charade.

Were PAPRs so cost prohibitive that they were worth more than the life of an anesthesiologist or intensivist or a respiratory therapist – $1300?!

Physicians in particular and many other healthcare personnel in general had started seeing through the CDC, DOH, AHA and many hospital systems guidance for masks and PPE, which was mainly due to shortage and for the purpose of rationing. The guidance was not for any altruistic purpose. It was neither meant to decrease transmission of COVID-19 nor was it for the primary purpose of safety of frontline healthcare personnel – the boots on the ground.

The AHA had already started lobbying congress, Speaker Nancy Pelosi, and Democrats "to withdraw workplace safety standards from a second package in response to the coronavirus pandemic." It appeared that the Republicans were approached as well for the same purpose of doing away of the safety standards.

Many physicians had started subscribing to the possibility based upon new studies that there was a high likelihood of airborne transmission of the virus in addition to the droplet and contact routes.

CDC, the DOH and many hospital systems still did not want hospital personnel to wear masks outside patient rooms. We had an increased but still manageable number of patients who were in isolation in COVID cohort units with adequate PPE and N95s so far. However, the number of patients who were suspicious, but not confirmed for COVID-19 as their COVID-19 tests were pending, were rising in number, necessitating more PPE requirement.

By March 19, 2020, CDC, which by then was on a downward spiral in terms of losing credibility, came up with the *bandana recommendation!*

COVIDSLAYERS

It recommended that healthcare personnel could use homemade scarves and bandanas to take care of COVID-19 patients instead of N95 and surgical masks if they are not available.

The CDC gave itself a disingenuous deniability stating that the capability of homemade masks to protect healthcare personnel is "unknown." We all know that it is not an unknown!

Bandanas, scarves, and even surgical masks do not provide adequate protection against aerosolized COVID-19 to the person wearing any one of them! It is the N95s that do!

N95 masks and other PPE are essential during patient care to not only prevent exposure to healthcare personnel from COVID-19 and other infections, but they are also supposed to be discarded after every patient interaction so that there is no transmission of COVID-19 and other infections from one patient to another and to other personnel. At least that was the recommendation as per CDC's own guidelines prior to mid–March 2020. Conventionally (everyday practice), they were/are also not supposed to be used beyond the manufacture designated shelf-life.

How would one as a patient feel if the gown that the nurse was wearing while taking care of that patient had been used by the nurse while taking care of 4 or 5 other patients?! Not to mention the predicament of the nurse who had to wear the same gown throughout the day for almost 12 hours while taking care of all those patients. It just sounds gross and disgusting. And thoughts about the anguish that the nurses would experience, day in and day out, almost makes one indignant at their predicament.

In addition, CDC also came up with another disingenuous recommendation saying, "health care providers exposed to coronavirus – even those who show mild symptoms – may also be advised to wear a face mask and continue treating patients."

Instead of recommending that these nurses and doctors boost their immunity, get sleep and rest, especially since there is no known cure, these nurses and doctors were now expected to work through their "mild" illness until they crashed with the dreaded cytokine storm, intubated and placed on a ventilator, in isolation, and away from their family. The family would

Dr. Rajesh Mohan

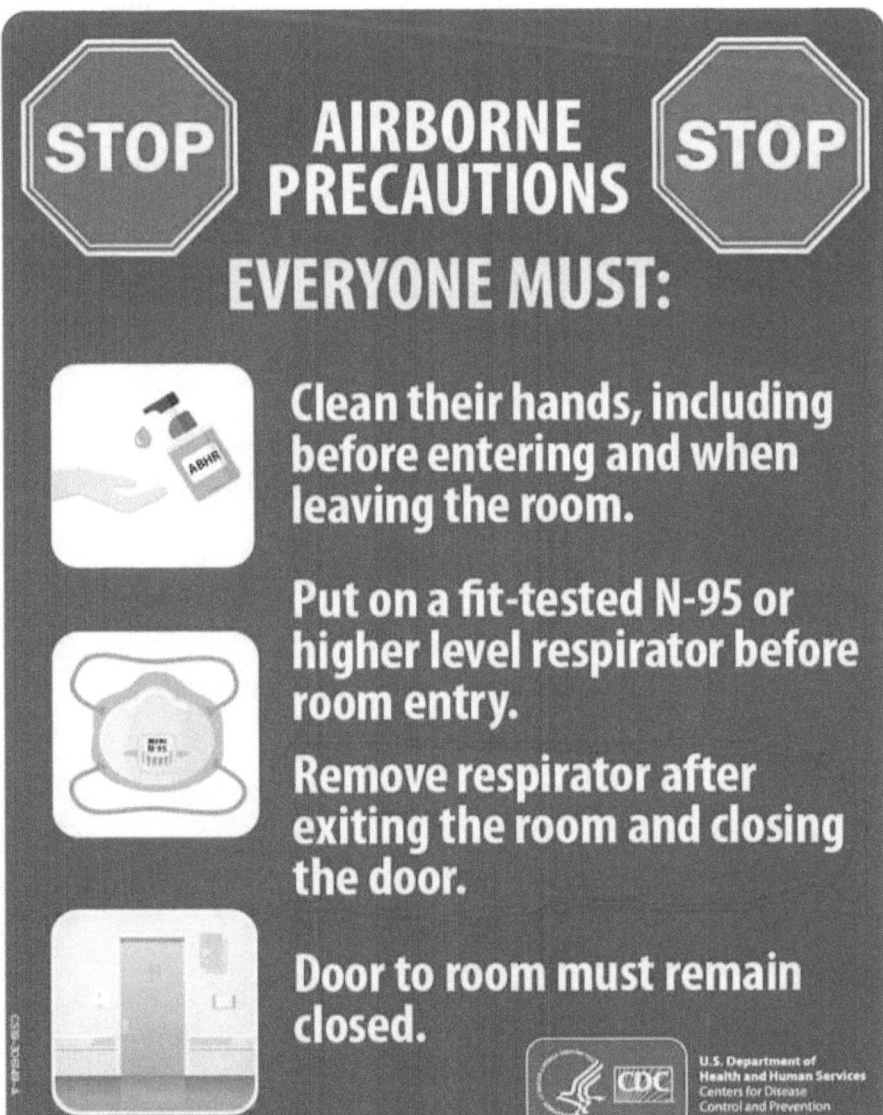

COVIDSLAYERS

 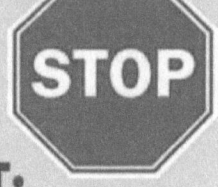

CONTACT PRECAUTIONS EVERYONE MUST:

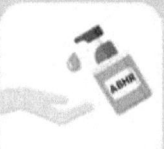 Clean their hands, including before entering and when leaving the room.

PROVIDERS AND STAFF MUST ALSO:

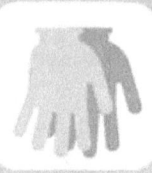 Put on gloves before room entry. Discard gloves before room exit.

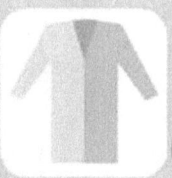 Put on gown before room entry. Discard gown before room exit.

Do not wear the same gown and gloves for the care of more than one person.

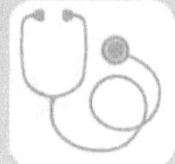 Use dedicated or disposable equipment. Clean and disinfect reusable equipment before use on another person.

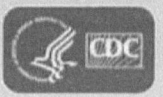 U.S. Department of Health and Human Services
Centers for Disease Control and Prevention

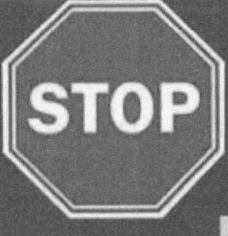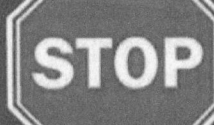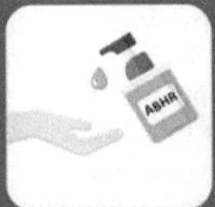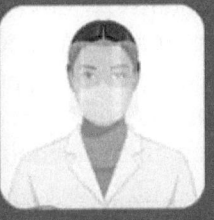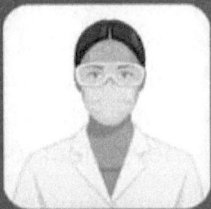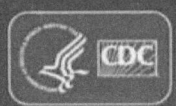

then pray and hope that their loved ones survive and do not end up becoming martyrs. Or they could get lucky and soldier on.

Healthcare entities using the CDC as a shield, in addition to having a callous disregard for the safety of nurses, physicians and other healthcare personnel, disingenuously disregarded the fact that these healthcare personnel could also be putting their families at risk as well as the patients and co-workers whom they would be coming in contact with. This not only had the potential for more tragic deaths including those of more patients and healthcare personnel but could also cause more propagation of the virus.

Physicians knew the difference between different masks and their ability to protect against the virus. N95 masks prevent the wearer from getting infected and should be worn when treating patients with infections, especially those like COVID-19 and tuberculosis. Surgical masks protect other people if the wearer has an infection but do not adequately protect the wearer from another person's infections, especially those like COVID-19 and tuberculosis. Guidelines were becoming a hazard to employee safety and a safe work environment in a war against an indiscriminate, invisible, and hostile enemy.

As medical professionals, we did not see "guidelines" change so frequently and so drastically, some almost daily. Many "guidelines" did not even make any sense, some being incoherent and some contradictory. Some were indefensible! Guidelines were becoming an impediment to critical thinking as well as creative thinking, which is what is required when one is dealing with the unknown, that too at such an overwhelming scale.

The CDC had started making a precipitous decline in its standards, recommendations, guidance and ultimately what would be, its credibility.

By Friday, March 20, 2020, it was becoming increasingly evident to the boots on the ground – doctors and nurses, specifically – that the CDC and the DOH had become irrelevant for the most part, especially regarding recommendations and guidelines that affected the healthcare personnel on how to interact with and manage COVID-19 patients. The CDC was floundering frequently. Administrators, healthcare policymakers and bureaucracies were taking disadvantage of the floundering CDC to justify their own agendas and incompetence. With more and more suspected COVID-19 patients admitted to hospitals, exposure to an increasing number of healthcare personnel in New York and in north New Jersey, and an increase in the number of infections in the community, it was apparent that community spread was becoming a reality.

The bandana recommendation and the recommendation to ask "mildly" sick healthcare personnel to continue to work with a mask on, pretty much shut the door on the CDC.

The CDC will have to get its act together soon, and there needs to be a revamping of the organization with not only qualified, but more importantly, competent scientists and physicians.

Most, if not all, hospitals and hospital organizations regularly gave daily updates and parroted the floundering CDC's guidelines.

However, it was heartening to notice that many of these updates from the CDC were ignored or interpreted differently by some local hospital clinical leaders and many clinicians. The physicians and nurses, for the most part, and a few clinical leaders and some clinical administrators who were not working from their offices but were actually seeing COVID-19 patients and working shoulder to shoulder with the boots on the ground, followed the science and utilized their critical thinking and decision-making skills for the benefit of patients and their fellow team members. Some did so more than others.

Based upon science and safety principles and concerns, some clinical physician administrative leaders decided to ride against the prevalent recommendations which were mainly based upon finance and expense reduction principles. These bold and brave leaders decided that it was time to act to protect the hospital staff rather than wait and potentially expose them to tragic consequences.

The message about adherence to best practice recommendations regarding hand hygiene, physical distancing and keeping work areas clean, especially with an apparent increase in community spread continued to be stressed. In addition, starting Friday, March 20, 2020, clinical physician

COVIDSLAYERS

leaders at many hospitals decided to proceed to practicing universal masking.

Now, healthcare personnel could wear masks outside patient rooms, thereby significantly decreasing their risk of exposure to the virus. All healthcare personnel continued to be reminded by clinical leaders at various hospitals – some more than others – to discard masks and PPE upon leaving an isolation room, including any COVID-19 isolation room.

It was time to do the right thing – even if it meant not believing the CDC's often changing modifications in their recommendations anymore!

As a result of universal masking and making sure that the hospital staff had adequate N95 masks and other PPE, many hospitals saw a significantly low hospital staff exposure rates to COVID-19.

Dr. Rajesh Mohan

Chapter Five

Science and Logic Became Dispensable

Very soon, it became abundantly evident that there was inadequate planning at best, and policies and guidance from the so-called higher levels in healthcare continued to be made on the fly. It was also apparent that the policymakers and administrators at various healthcare entities, for the most part, appeared to be lost and did not know what they were doing. The frequent and common use by administrators and people in power and policy-making positions of ambivalent statements and phrases such as – "I/we don't know," "we will try to figure it out," "we are working on it" were rarely heard so often when faced with a crisis situation.

In addition, healthcare personnel who were at the forefront of the onslaught and fighting the battle – boots on the ground – were being asked and expected to wait and stay in limbo. And, when the uninspiring so-called "guidelines" were eventually being released, and many times in a piecemeal approach, all healthcare personnel were expected to adhere to them as rules until the next couple of days or so, when the so-called guidelines would be modified again.

To add to the lackadaisical approach, some supply chain and "safety" operations personnel were either not aware of the national emergency stockpile or even if they were aware of such an entity, had not contacted their local Office of Emergency Management (OEM). Even the OEM officials appeared to be frustrated at the lack of anticipation for expected needs such as N95 masks, PPE, or ventilators, and the lack of preparedness for emergency situations by most healthcare entities, as well as the sluggish approach by key stakeholders.

I believe administrators at many hospitals, however, were quick to anticipate and plan in advance the hoarding or "sequestering" of N95 masks and other PPE in the days and weeks prior to the onslaught of the pandemic so as to be able to ration their use by the very people who would be in contact with patients and therefore need them the most – nurses, doctors and hospital staff.

Insinuations and sometimes accusations at various hospitals were being made unashamedly by non-clinical supply chain personnel and some administrators, that nurses and doctors would "steal" PPE if they were left in places where they had usually been kept for years.

This hoarding or "sequestration" of essential PPE by administrators led to a perception of a higher level of scarcity and panic leading to more hoarding. As a result, essential PPE was being kept out of reach and easy access from essential clinical healthcare personnel. Anguished healthcare personnel who were in direct contact with patients and needed PPE the most were being given impossible choices. The same disposable masks, gloves and gowns which were supposed to be discarded after being used for one patient to avoid carrying and transmitting infections from one patient to another as well as to other team members, were now expected to be used by nurses and doctors and other direct patient-care giving healthcare personnel, for an entire day and with multiple patients.

By March 2020, in many hospitals masks and PPE were hoarded or "sequestered" by administrators and supply chain personnel. Therefore, they were not available outside patient rooms like they used to be. With widespread rationing of PPE and the rising fear of COVID-19, many healthcare personnel were led toward confusion and difficult choices about how to best utilize the limited number of rationed masks and PPE that they were being provided.

COVIDSLAYERS

It would have been a different story if the supply chain personnel and financial administrators had simply done their job. They could have easily procured enough N95 masks and PPE in January and February 2020 when the alarm bells were ringing loud and clear of an advancing *infectious disease* pandemic. Even the prices were cheaper then. Masks that used to be sold for $0.58 were now being sold for $7 dollars per unit. If they were concerned enough to anticipate a shortage leading them to hoard N95s and PPE, then the same concerns could and should have been channeled in a positive rather than a negative direction. A positive approach would have then led them to procuring and creating a stockpile of N95 masks and other PPE for at least a three to six-month supply, instead of hoarding. They obviously did not.

It was also a penny-wise pound-foolish strategy, as even the least competent financial administrator and supply chain personnel must know that prices go up when supply is less and demand is high in a free market economy, in the absence of any price caps. It was only a matter of time before the same people would be forced to spend more money for the same products.

Although they may now shed crocodile tears and sympathize with lip service for the trauma that was caused to healthcare personnel as a result, these administrators and non-clinical supply chain personnel were essentially forced to eventually spend *more* money than they would have otherwise done. They apparently had no choice, mainly due to a rising hue and cry in the media and among nursing staff, hospital staff and physicians, regarding the lack of PPE provided to frontline healthcare personnel which in many cases possibly even resulted in deaths of healthcare personnel.

Given the fact that N95 masks and other PPE would be essential to protect hospital staff while they were taking care of patients, it was obvious that a ramp up of N95 mask and PPE supply was urgently needed. Most entities including the OEM were providing essential PPE to hospitals on a first come first serve basis.

It was becoming apparent that it was going to be a *survival of the fittest*.

Due to continued increased delays in the turnaround times of COVID-19 tests with major "contracted" laboratories, some physician healthcare leaders utilized their entrepreneurial skills and knowledge about the marketplace in finding alternate vendors who would process these tests with a better turnaround time. However, even the best turnaround times for COVID-19 results available were still between 2-4 days – not ideal, but better than the turnaround time of 4–7 days at major "contracted" laboratories.

Availability of COVID-19 tests with rapid turnaround time are inextricably linked to PPE and particularly N95 usage. The situation was worsened due to delay in results of COVID-19 tests which resulted in an increased usage of limited PPE as hospital staff could not presume that patients whose tests were pending were COVID-19 negative and therefore they had to use the already rationed PPE during any patient interaction until the results were back.

It has always frustrated doctors and nurses that the administrators and politicians find it so hard to understand and accept (either intentionally or unintentionally) the concept that PPE usage and COVID-19 tests are directly linked.

If COVID-19 tests are readily available with a rapid turnaround time, then the PPE usage shrinks significantly. Both of these basic components were, and still are, essential if we want to contain the COVID-19 pandemic. There cannot be any cutting of corners in the procurement and availability of these two basic necessities. Any compromise on these two basic necessities will continue to have negative consequences and create hurdles in the fight against the COVID-19 pandemic.

It was exasperating that despite an abysmal shortage of COVID-19 tests, healthcare administrators and politicians touted testing availability with statements such as those from the Health Commissioner of New Jersey on March 17th stating, "I don't believe anyone who needs the test is not getting it." Many doctors, nurses and many from the public were dismayed when they heard this statement. Some wondered where the Health Commissioner was getting the information from, or whether such statements were just made up and delivered cavalierly.

COVIDSLAYERS

An apt eye-opener for the public health officials came very soon in the form of the first drive-through testing center which was finally opened at the end of the week on Friday, March 20, 2020. This would be overwhelmed immediately, reaching capacity within four hours. Other drive through centers would eventually open in the weeks to come, delayed mainly due to bureaucratic inefficiencies, poor planning, and incompetence.

Some administrators at several healthcare entities continue to give excuses that they did not expect "it" to be so bad. These administrators and policymakers, if they still do say this and continue to use this as an excuse for having kept their heads in the sand, should be educated and counseled regarding their incompetence and arrogance, which could have been bolstered by their own insecurities. However, if this rationale is being used disingenuously by them so as to absolve themselves of any responsibility despite the tragedies that have occurred, then their persistence in a public service based healthcare institution may result in further negative repercussions to patients, dedicated healthcare personnel and healthcare in general.

Disingenuously and unabashedly, some other administrators have now even started to state audaciously but falsely, that they were and have been able to provide adequate supply of N95 masks and other PPE, in an effort to hide their incompetence and re-write history. This perverse and dishonest behavior has surfaced even while N95 masks and PPE are still being rationed and reprocessing of disposable, one-time use N95 masks is still being enforced by administrators while hiding behind inadequate science, and at best guidance from CDC that pertains to contingency (expected shortages) and crisis (known shortages) capacity scenarios. So far, there have been no significant peer reviewed randomized control trials comparing exposure risk to COVID-19 with one-time N95 mask use versus N95 masks that have been reprocessed multiple times especially when used continuously for more than 12 hours (usually one shift).

About nine months into the pandemic there must not be any contingency and crisis scenarios regarding N95 masks and other PPE procurement and availability. The body armor required in the fight against this pandemic must be readily and easily available to the healthcare warriors on the frontline.

After more than nine months of the initial COVID-19 assault on the people of this country which the American healthcare personnel so valiantly continue to fight against, if hospitals and healthcare agencies are still in a contingency or a crisis mode regarding body armor – N95 masks and other PPE – that they are morally and duty bound to provide to their healthcare warriors, then there are bigger systemic as well as ethical problems in our healthcare system's administration than those that have been exposed even by this pandemic.

At the very least, it was and is the cost of doing business!

COVIDSLAYERS

Dr. Rajesh Mohan

Chapter Six

Misplaced Priorities

Healthcare Is About Patients First, Stupid!

Other than issues related to PPE and COVID-19 tests, there were additional issues brewing and some started to surface.

There were reports coming in that in New York, due to potential shortage of ventilators, a rationing of ventilators was being contemplated – which would mean that physicians may have to choose which patient would be intubated and placed on a ventilator in case of limited availability of ventilators. There were reports that terminal extubations were either being contemplated or were being carried out in New York.

There was also concern expressed by many, including in the local community, asking if we would be holding back on intubations and cardiopulmonary resuscitations (CPR) and potentially let patients die if they were critically sick. The same concern began rising among physicians as well, which was, if they would be forced into the same predicament and have to make those unfortunate and tragic decisions.

Hospitals over Patients?!

Most policymakers and administrators were worried about overwhelming the hospitals. Many thought that hospitals would not have enough beds, especially ICU beds to take care of patients.

Patients were being advised to go to the ER or hospitals only if they were severely sick. Patients who were mildly sick or were able to get care staying home were asked to stay home so that the hospitals were not overwhelmed.

In addition, the Centers for Medicare and Medicaid Services (CMS) decided to waive the requirement of a 3-day hospitalization prior to being transferred to a skilled nursing facility (SNF) – except CMS probably did not realize that SNFs had the challenge of PPE availability as well, and therefore, regardless of the waiver, would not accept COVID-19 patients and take the risk of spreading COVID-19 to their elderly and high risk residents. Therefore, SNFs started to require patients in hospitals to have COVID-19 tests that needed to be negative prior to accepting patients.

And yes, COVID-19 test results still were not coming back until 4–7 days. Consequently, the waiver of a 3-day hospitalization requirement did not really matter or help much at that time. Patients who could not go home continued to stay in the hospital waiting for COVID-19 test results to be negative.

To add to the tragic bewilderment at the incoherent policies to "protect" the overwhelming of hospitals was a memo from the Office of the Chief State Medical Examiner, mis-dated as 3/25/19 instead of 3/25/20, stating that "for hospital cases that have outstanding COVID-19 tests if there is an established diagnosis (e.g. pneumonia) the case can be released and the treating physician should list the cause of death as 'Pending COVID-19 testing', with a natural manner of death. They will need to issue an amendment once test results are received. This should ease delays in burial." Except that the state probably was unaware that many funeral homes were not accepting dead bodies until there was a confirmation of COVID-19 test – negative or positive.

Interestingly, but tragically, most, if not all, policymakers and administrators who always worked hard to try to fill their hospital beds to make money, were now all of a sudden more worried about hospitals being overwhelmed.

Sadly, they were not thinking about the patients and the general public.

The administrators primary concern was that hospitals would become overwhelmed. They were not as much concerned about the virus overwhelming the patients or the public and certainly were not terribly concerned about the possibility of a rapid spread of the disease. It would be the rapid spread of disease that would overwhelm hospitals!

They were thinking backwards!

If only greater efforts had been directed towards containment of the disease, educating the public to wear masks, physical distancing, and hand hygiene. More importantly, if hospitals had set up testing centers in coordination with local communities, identifying asymptomatic patients and providing early management (even supportive) to symptomatic patients with recommendations of self-isolation and contact tracing and with that taking care of patients earlier rather than later, we probably would have been in a much better place and fewer people would have died. Hospital beds could have been added simultaneously which were being done anyway.

It should have been patients first – not hospitals first! It should always be that way!

Were the sick members of the general public not supposed to seek medical attention when they thought that they needed to? Were they supposed to let their condition worsen and possibly even die at home? Or were they supposed to show up in the hospital ER when they were on death's door?

In addition, the policymakers and administrators did not apparently either realize or understand that these mildly or moderately sick COVID-19 patients, while at home, would be spreading COVID-19 without any guided or recommended self-isolation.

What, if any, logical or medical sense did this all make?

Prevention is better than Cure

Numerous symptomatic individuals were unable to get COVID-19 tests which possibly undermined and hindered the state's ability to comprehend the full scope of the onslaught of the pandemic in the state of New Jersey as well as other places in the U.S.

The general public continued to get infected from these mildly and moderately symptomatic individuals in addition to the forty percent asymptomatic and pre-symptomatic COVID carriers. So, it did not make sense to not test more people – asymptomatic, mildly, and moderately symptomatic. The severely symptomatic were being tested when they showed up in the ER and were then admitted, some of whom then died.

The basic dictum of primary prevention, early recognition and management of disease, and the primary reason of why healthcare establishments are in existence, which is to take care of the sick – all of the above, was discarded and thrown out of the window.

The number of hospitalized patients and those patients who have died in a hospital from COVID-19, were and are known, as they get tested and counted. These numbers will keep increasing if infection from the virus spreads more – which would happen more if we do not know who has the virus and who is spreading the virus.

Therefore, more testing associated with self-isolation and coupled with contact tracing is essential if we want to defeat the virus.

Think about that for a few seconds!

Whether more people get tested or not – if more people are infected, then more people get sick, which leads to more people dying. Patients who are hospitalized and the patients who die especially in a hospital are counted anyway. If we do not test the asymptomatic or mildly asymptomatic who do not need hospitalization and do not die, they then keep infecting others, some of whom would then end up in a hospital and some of them would die. The virus would keep spreading and people would keep getting sick and dying. It is tragic. It can be avoided!

Therefore, more COVID tests are needed so that people who are identified as positive are then placed in isolation for 14 days so that they do not infect others – which then results in less number of people getting infected leading to less number of people getting sick which would lead to less number of people dying.

It should really not be that difficult to understand. It should not be made complicated!

The number of patients with suspected COVID-19 being admitted to hospitals was steadily increasing. Test results continued to have increased delays. Many symptomatic patients who were not sick enough to go to the hospital were unable to get tested for COVID-19. In addition to limited availability and long turnaround times for COVID tests, people were also unable to get tests due to strict criteria as per the limited and short-sighted initial and changing CDC guidelines. Testing guidelines were being made, not based upon science, but instead upon the concept of rationing, just like PPE.

Clinical acumen and clinical decision making were being coerced and sometimes forced to take a back seat in the thought process that was being utilized for policy making regarding public health and patient care, placing the general public in jeopardy. It was only at the end of April 2020 that NIH launched RADx to support the development, production scale up, and deployment of accurate, rapid tests across the country after the US Congress appropriated $1.5 billion on April 24th, 2020 to the NIH.

Just like PPE, if only the policymakers and administrators had not failed to anticipate and had made testing available in the weeks and months prior to the onslaught!

Suspected COVID-19 patients had started coming to the ER and some were admitted with their tests pending since admission. Physicians were asked to follow the CDC criteria for COVID-19 testing which was limited to symptomatic patients with a travel history to certain hot spots. A streamlined process to follow such criteria with twenty-four-hour access for testing was established. However, the tests were not done in-house and were sent out – turnaround time for results was not in the hands of physicians.

All surgeries and procedures, unless medically necessary, were postponed. In many hospitals, the Chair of Surgery and the Chair of Anesthesia were assigned the responsibility to review all surgeries and procedures prior to proceeding with any surgery. Going forward and until the initial surge subsided, they would be screening all such patients day and night, as well as the weekends. Only emergent and urgent surgeries that were assessed and deemed as such and necessary were going to be performed.

Outpatient hospital services were being wound down in preparation for the rising tide of COVID-19 patients. Similarly, many hospitals had assigned the Chair of Radiology to screen all radiology procedures for necessity mainly due to restricted and limited availability of N95 masks and other PPE and to decrease the risk of exposure, transmission, and propagation of the virus.

Patients were developing fear of going to hospitals. With policies placing severe restrictions and limitations on visitors, patients were afraid of getting admitted to any hospital as they did not want to be there alone and unable to see a loved one with no chance of being visited by a family member during their stay with some exceptions under extreme circumstances.

Dr. Rajesh Mohan

All these policies of restrictions were based upon and mainly due to mostly actual and some perceived shortage of resources that included N95 masks and other PPE, absence of adequate number of rapid COVID-19 tests, as well as limitation of nursing and critical care staff and critical care hospital supplies and beds.

Did any policymaker or administrator even think about patients as their top priority? Were patients really their top priority when they sat down in board rooms to deliberate and prepare for the pandemic? Since when did restriction and denial of patient care and patient care services become one of the initial items for policy making and implementation in healthcare?

If only the policymakers and administrators had really prepared when there was time, with patients as their top priority, rather than having to rush through at the last minute.

This was not preparation. This was a cop-out!

What would happen to patients with heart disease, cancer, stroke, kidney failure and other medical conditions that may require hospitalization, especially since many outpatient doctors' offices were being shut down due to the rising tide of COVID-19 associated with the lack of PPE, N95 masks and COVID-19 tests?

Adding to the confusion, state and multiple other agencies soon started demanding data from hospitals using their own varied definitions. Many hospitals started grappling with changing their data collection methodologies so as to conform to the requirements of different agencies.

Even a simple exercise of data collection was neither planned nor synchronized by all these so-called high-powered agencies and regulatory bureaucratic behemoths, resulting in chaos and waste of precious time of the hospital staff that could have been utilized in a more efficient and productive manner.

Many times, it appeared that there were certain administrators who were simply pushing paper and coming up with changing definitions and requirements just for the sole purpose of maintaining their job security while wasting other people's time.

COVIDSLAYERS

It was so hard to believe that in this age of technology, manual data entry was still being utilized by these colossal entities that were supposed to be leaders in and of healthcare.

There were reports that many COVID-19 patients were neither being diagnosed nor counted, many of them getting better and some of them dying.

If Johns Hopkins University could have a running dashboard for the entire world, then was it so difficult to collect and maintain real-time data locally and within a state?

In the midst of all this bureaucratic mess, I received an invitation for a conference on behalf of the Centers for Medicare and Medicaid Services (CMS) with the main topics, believe it or not, being –

Put Patients Over Paperwork!

Increase Hospital Capacity – CMS Hospitals Without Wall

Rapidly Expand the Healthcare Workforce

Further Promote Telehealth in Medicare!

Dr. Rajesh Mohan

CMS "OFFICE HOURS" ON COVID-19

The IPRO QIN QIO is forwarding this information on behalf of the Centers for Medicare & Medicaid Services (CMS)

You are invited to CMS "Office Hours" on COVID-19, Thursday, April 16° from 5:00 – 6:00 PM EST, the next in a series of opportunities for hospitals, health systems, and providers to ask questions of agency officials regarding CMS's temporary actions that empower local hospitals and healthcare systems to:

- Increase Hospital Capacity – CMS Hospitals Without Walls;
- Rapidly Expand the Healthcare Workforce;
- Put Patients Over Paperwork; and
- Further Promote Telehealth in Medicare

We encourage you to submit questions in advance to partnership@cms.hhs.gov, including "Office Hours" in the subject line. There will also be live Q&A

Dial in details are below:

Toll-Free Attendee Dial In: ▇▇▇▇▇▇▇▇

Event Plus Passcode: ▇▇▇▇▇▇

Audio Webcast link: ▇▇▇▇▇▇▇▇▇▇▇▇▇▇▇▇▇▇▇▇▇▇▇▇

Conference lines are limited, so we highly encourage you to join via audio webcast, either on your computer or smartphone web browser.

You are welcome to share this invitation with your colleagues and membership. These actions, and earlier CMS actions in response to COVID-19, are part of the ongoing White House Coronavirus Task Force efforts. To keep up with the important work the Task Force is doing in response to COVID-19, visit www.coronavirus.gov. For a complete and updated list of CMS actions, and other information specific to CMS, please visit the Current Emergencies Website.

Click here for full press release and related materials

COVIDSLAYERS

It appeared that in the vast swamp of our unhealthy healthcare system, someone woke up and had an epiphany!

Our unhealthy healthcare system and its administrators have immense power to sway the mighty and the righteous into crossing over to the dark side. If they are so powerful that they can manipulate healthcare as they choose for their own benefit, while influencing the lives of all Americans frequently enough in a negative way, what are the chances any individual will have in affecting change – I thought.

Would it not have made more sense if certain hospitals across the state at strategic locations were designated as COVID-19 hospitals? – I said to myself.

Management of COVID patients, data collection and monitoring of COVID patients would then have been seamless. Resources such as COVID-19 tests, N95 masks and other PPE, and medications could have been allocated and utilized in a more efficient manner instead of them being scattered across all hospitals – big and small – across the state with inefficient use and distribution.

Physicians and nurses – the boots on the ground – had been pleading for preparedness. We knew it was too late now and that no matter what anyone tried to justify it with – we were not prepared. Now, there was no option but to play catch up.

Politicians can always be blamed, and most are rightly so. However, it is their so-called advisors, experts, policymakers, and administrators who really failed BIG-TIME. Politicians, with exceptions, for the most part are only as good as their advisors, who can speak truth to power and do not hedge, especially about consequential matters.

This is a once in a lifetime and a once-in-a-100-year pandemic! People's lives were and still are at stake.

A thorough robust response to the pandemic with fewer lives lost should have been the only option.

If for nothing else, this would have benefited the administrative and political careers of administrators and advisors. In addition, it would have benefited the fortunes of their political masters. They would have benefited if they were up to their jobs. It has been nothing else but sheer incompetence of opportunistic people holding onto positions of power where they had no business being in the first place. They have not only failed at their jobs and their political masters, but more importantly, they have failed the very people who they had been hired to serve – the American people.

If COVID-19 tests and test results could have been made available in a timely manner, patients could then be asked to seek medical attention earlier rather than later.

If adequate PPE were made available for healthcare personnel to perform tests and while taking care of patients – many decisions such as SNF waiver would have been a success.

If PPE and COVID-19 tests were more readily available, more doctors' offices would have been able to take care of patients with early identification and self-isolation instead of having to shut down.

Instead of not venturing out of their homes until they were so sick that they had to go to the hospital, patients could have and should have been able to seek medical attention sooner before they got caught in the dreaded cytokine storm leading them to the ER, and in many cases, death.

Made up Treatment "Protocols" and "Algorithms"

In the early days of the pandemic reaching New Jersey, pharmacists driven so-called treatment protocols and algorithms were being sent to physicians treating and managing COVID-19 patients on the frontlines in various hospitals. These so-called treatment protocols and algorithms presumptuously did not have any significant input from physician leaders or Department Chiefs who were the ones who were devising treatment strategies on the frontlines. In addition, brazen demands that physicians follow these pretentious algorithms were being made.

COVIDSLAYERS

Many physicians found it laughable that while there was no known proven treatment available for COVID-19, some pharmacists, most likely at the behest of administrators along with one or more physician "sponsor(s)" or "champion(s)," had manufactured a treatment protocol which they now wanted the treating physicians to adhere to. A physician "sponsor" or "champion" is usually a physician (most often an employed physician who is promoted as an expert) who would usually acquiesce with minimal resistance if any, and is used by administrators to further their agendas and policies with some ascribed level of credibility to make them acceptable to physicians at large.

In the minds of many physicians, this was apparently being done by administrators in many hospitals with the same thought process they applied to N95 masks and PPE – which was to hoard or "sequester" medications so as to be able to ration them as well. Was it about money-over-patients, as is in many instances? Was it their incompetence in procuring commonly available medications and a few new medications?

Needless to say, and not surprisingly, the so-called treatment protocol was not even given a second thought by many physicians. The so-called treatment protocol was given the same treatment by most physicians as one of the multitudes of junk emails that were being sent, mostly by administrators and personnel sitting in offices who, for the most part, had no direct clinical contact with COVID-19 patients and who were, for the most part, not actively managing COVID-19 patients on the frontlines.

It appears that this pandemic has revealed one of the worst traits of bureaucracies and those that are associated with administrative process related inertia – the propensity to do the least possible.

This minimalistic behavior was evident even when community organizations wanted to donate medications and supplies to hospitals to replenish shortages of medications and supplies that many were acutely aware of. Offers of donating expensive medications and vitamins that were legitimate and approved by regulatory agencies were met by negativity, skepticism and even cynicism by administrators in bureaucracies in hospitals. This negativity occurred in the guise of "unproven medical treatment for COVID-19" or assumptions of spurious medications before a vetting process would be even started.

Physicians have always wondered what was the rationale, if any? Or was it that they were just lazy that they had to do paperwork and verification of the donation and then stock it in the pharmacy? Did it ever come across in their minds that this could potentially benefit patients? Were they even thinking about the patients?

Even if this would have happened under normal circumstances and not during a pandemic, one is forced to wonder – whatever happened to common sense?

Social Media and the COVID-19 Medical Community

Meanwhile, physicians who were in the forefront were actively making clinical management decisions which had life and death consequences for patients whom they had the responsibility to take care of. This included trying medications and treatment modalities as long as they were safe, even though they may have been experimental and off-label. This was in addition to supportive treatment based upon the clinical presentation and subsequent course of the disease process and the patient's condition.

In the absence of any definitive well-established and effective treatments, physicians were relying upon each other locally, as well as on national and international physician communities. They were learning from studies and experiences in earlier COVID-19 exposed areas such as California, Washington, New York, Italy, and China. Management strategies for COVID-19 patients was also derived from the medical knowledge that we all (physicians) attain in medical school about topics, that among others, included infections, immunology, multiorgan system failure, inflammatory processes, epidemiology, as well as how to manage pandemics. Treatments were also based upon the experiences of physicians within the local community as well as physicians practicing in different academic centers and community hospitals in the U.S.

COVIDSLAYERS

There was an increased level of communication and an open and uninhibited exchange of thought processes among physicians at a personal level, as well as in social media, with groups having been formed that were dedicated to learning about and management of COVID-19.

There were apolitical physician groups pertaining to COVID-19 that had sprung up on social media. Many physicians had stopped going to the hospitals as well as closed their offices. Most patients did not venture out of their homes leading to closed doctors' offices. Most patients in the hospital were COVID-19 patients, and therefore there was less of a requirement for many physician specialties. Many physicians belonging to such less required specialties were, however, active on social media. They were following, contributing, and collecting information regarding COVID-19 in statewide groups and nationwide groups, as well as international groups.

With the benefit of cutting edge knowledge and information, many physicians in these social media groups were challenging hospitals and hospital administrators throughout the country and sparking movements and pressurizing hospitals to provide adequate PPE for the protection of their fellow physicians and nurses who were on the front lines.

In addition, different clinical experiences and practices were shared among physicians locally, statewide, nationally, and internationally. Most scientific studies and data were shared on these social media sites much earlier than other forums, after which followed a robust peer review almost in real-time. The New Jersey COVID-19 Physician/APP Facebook group had about 600 members. The COVID-19 USA Physician/APP Facebook group had about 150,000 members! These groups had robust, updated, and apolitical information with real-time peer review of studies, data, and clinical practice recommendations regarding the pandemic.

This organic organization of numerous physicians along with the information and interactions within these groups substantially helped frontline physician colleagues. The vacuum created by the mostly absent state and national physician organizations was filled seamlessly, effectively, and more efficiently by these groups. In addition to improvements in the care of COVID-19 patients, the information, and interactions within these groups helped in making sure that the hospital administrators were given reality checks time and again–sometimes with tangible results.

Financial Administrators and Healthcare

The number of COVID-19 patients continued to rise in hospitals throughout the state of NJ. More units were being converted into COVID units. The number of COVID-19 patients requiring ICU care was steadily increasing as well. Appropriate and adequate critical care nurse staffing need was becoming even more urgent. Respiratory therapists had begun experiencing burn out. Requests for additional respiratory therapists remained pending. Tangible actions and results from administrators responsible for ensuring adequate staffing were victims of bureaucratic inertia and glacial thought processes.

The wheels of "financial" administrators were still dragging – 2 weeks into the initial surge of the pandemic in many hospitals. It was apparent that with bureaucratic inertia, even the procurement of adequate number of critical care nurses was becoming a survival of the fittest. Pleas were being made by physicians, nurses and even politicians on television for healthcare personnel in other parts of the country to come to NY and NJ to help their fellow colleagues. They were ready, but someone had to pay them. Who would that be?

Anticipating the inertia and the glacial pace that is prevalent in the thinking and operation of financial administrators in healthcare, nursing leadership had been providing additional education and training to improve competencies of nurses and technicians from other departments within the hospital. This was initiated to establish patient care delivery models and assist nurses in critical care and medical telemetry units due to a shortage of such nurses. Nurses are nurses – they do not shy away from taking care of patients even if it means just-in-time training and a steep learning curve which may be required to be able to provide patient care in areas with complexities that they may not be accustomed to.

COVIDSLAYERS

Almost all hospitals in the tri-state area were vying for resources, which included critical care nurses. Physicians and physician leaders knew the critical role of and need for ICU nurses required for adequate patient care. In addition to critical care nurses with more COVID-19 patients who required critical care, there was a growing requirement of physicians, including intensivists and anesthesiologists.

It was apparent that when NY and NJ hospitals had reached the crisis point, and not before, "financial" administrators finally acquiesced to approving more physician staff, including intensivists and critical nurses. However, as the decision was made when hospitals had already reached the crisis mode and not before (unfortunately for the purpose to save money), the challenge was to find additional physicians, nurses and respiratory therapists who were willing to immerse themselves into this pandemic. In addition, they were now at a premium, even if someone was lucky in finding them. Penny wise, pound foolish – once again. If only the planning and procurement was done earlier!

How is it even justified for financial administrators to have so much of an influence and authority in determining what level of physician and nurse staffing would provide adequate patient care? – physicians have often wondered.

Physicians, nurses, and respiratory therapists are not items that sit on shelves such that they can simply be picked up for use when one decides to do so. It takes time to secure them, as they are not mere inanimate objects in an assembly line – they have families and other responsibilities. They are humans!

Why would anyone, anyone go *small* in a pandemic, *any pandemic*? – I have asked, many times.

Dr. Rajesh Mohan

Chapter Seven

Bigotry and Humanity–In a Pandemic

Most hospitals were in a lockdown phase with suspended patient visitation rights, leaving admitted patients bereft of the opportunity to be comforted by their loved ones.

While nurses and physicians were doing their best to keep family members informed, those efforts were limited in scope and occurrences. By the end of March and early April 2020, many sick COVID-19 patients who had recovered from their acute illness were ready for discharge from hospitals. However, due to lingering post-COVID symptoms, many required supplemental oxygen and oxygen concentrators at home – which were in limited supply. In addition, hospitals were unable to procure these supplies for an alarming number of patients who did not have medical insurance. If these patients were not able to be provided with home oxygen, they could not be safely discharged, given the strong likelihood of them returning to the emergency room, possibly in a worse condition. These circumstances led to hospital stays being extended longer than otherwise necessary for many patients, all while they were being separated from their family and loved ones.

With growing public awareness of this predicament, certain philanthropic and local religious organizations made efforts to assuage the situation. When made aware of this predicament, local community organizations, like the New Jersey based nonprofit organization *Bikur Cholim*, stepped up without hesitation and provided these essentials to patients at no cost so the patients could complete their recovery safely at home with their families and, perhaps as importantly, free-up much needed hospital beds for the onslaughts of patients.

There were also many discussions taking place across the country with local community leaders of the possibility of hiring patient liaisons with medical knowhow from certain demographically relevant minority communities, who could serve as an intermediary between medical and nursing staff and ALL patient families, and *also* meaningfully fill the void felt by patients of certain religious and ethnic persuasions. Many in the medical and local communities believed that such a liaison would serve multiple roles. Not only would they free up the medical team from providing more frequent updates, but would also be able to coordinate with the treating physicians and nurses to communicate relevant medical information to the families of patients in a manner that was sensitive to the religious practices and beliefs of certain communities, where relevant. This form of enriched communication could provide the patient and their families an additional level of comfort and confidence regarding the care being administered to their loved ones.

While many of my colleagues were successful in forging such relationships and implementing such a program, shockingly, some received significant bureaucratic pushback. I came to understand that while certain administrators were quite vocal against such hiring, others guised it by a deft combination of obfuscation and red tape – a skill often ubiquitous among those adept in the art of maintaining job security.

Was it that some administrators did not want to spend money? Did they believe that the mental and emotional well-being of patients and their families did not have much value? Was it possible that the resistance was because the person was from a different faith? Some questions and mindsets that need exploring. Thankfully, however, the senior leadership of many other hospitals, including mine, agreed and understood the immediate positive and beneficial impact that a liaison would bring.

COVIDSLAYERS

Over the course of this pandemic, much attention has been, and continues to be, directed by the media toward certain ethnic and religious groups. I do not believe this to be a systemic issue with our media, rather one that pervades all communities. We often tend to be drawn to the comfort of thinking in the binary. What appeals to our sensibilities even more is the shiftless demonization of a community we find easy not to identify with.

Despite many hospitals hiring liaisons, I came to believe that many such liaisons from Orthodox Jewish communities were, and continue to be, subjected to not-so-guised "othering." I believe it was not uncommon to read or hear comments such as: "they" are spreading the virus by having weddings and funerals and large gatherings; usage of the word "they" in a seemingly derogatory manner; references to religious practices and rituals with disrespect; and attempts at mockery or scorn in other instances.

Despite the obvious, it apparently does not occur to many people that the spread of the virus is not limited to one religion or community. There have been some people that belong to different religions, communities, age-groups, and social and educational backgrounds who have not, and continue to not, take the pandemic seriously.

There has been non-adherence to virus containment tactics such as wearing masks and physical distancing by groups of people from all backgrounds. People who do not follow recommended guidance at events and venues such as beaches, parties, political rallies, parks, and restaurants belong to all different faiths and backgrounds.

Generalizing, blaming, and harboring prejudice and intolerance toward any particular community or religion for the non-compliance by a few (like there are in any community), is bigotry. And, bigotry should have no place in society – not during a pandemic. Please!

I came to understand from physician friends and colleagues across the tri-state region that although patient liaisons were hired by hospitals to serve the needs of all patients regardless of their faith, incorrect assumptions were being made that they would *only* serve the Orthodox Jewish patient population. Skepticism and cynicism were automatically ascribed to this role. While to my knowledge, neither my colleagues at other hospitals, nor I am aware of any formal complaints highlighting this discrimination, I suspect the anti-Semitic statements and barely concealed bias inflicted on such communities across the country may very well become public knowledge over the course of time. And even if they do not, we as a society should take stock of our behavior. To paraphrase a recently made common phrase, a pandemic does not change who you are, it reveals who you are.

And who is this much maligned Orthodox Jewish Community? To provide some context, let me take you to the period toward the end of March when COVID-19 was running rampant through New York. There were reports that Mount Sinai Hospital in New York was considering convalescent plasma as a treatment modality for COVID-19 patients. Convalescent plasma had been used as a treatment modality in the past for similar viral illnesses and was studied during the H1N1 influenza virus pandemic of 2009-2010, 2003 SARS-CoV-1 epidemic, and the 2012 MERS-CoV epidemic.

However, to make the convalescent plasma even possible, there needed to be donors. Not just any donors, but those who had adequate level of antibodies to the virus that caused COVID-19. By April, although many people were infected and had recovered from COVID-19, there just were not enough donors with adequate levels of antibodies and therefore there was not enough plasma.

As per news reports, in one of the most audacious acts of humanity and leadership, the Jewish community in Lakewood, NJ was mobilized by Rabbi Yehudah Kaszirer, the Director of Lev Rochel Bikur Cholim of Lakewood, New Jersey, to come together at a moment's notice in mid-April 2020, resulting in the collection of 1,000 vials of blood within 24 hours. These vials, reportedly, were then stored in coolers, loaded by 3:00 A.M on a private jet, and delivered to the Mayo Clinic in Rochester, Minnesota by the Rabbi himself, so that they could then be tested for antibodies. As per news reports, soon after he was back in NJ that noon, the Rabbi started receiving results on the antibodies. Eligible donors were informed right away, who then proceeded to donating plasma starting the very next morning. It has been reported that roughly 60 percent or about 600 out of that initial collection of 1,000 vials of blood samples were found to contain antibodies. As per Dr. Michael J. Joyner, who leads the Mayo Clinic's plasma program, "since that overnight flight, Orthodox Jews in Kaszirer's community and others across the country have provided an extraordinary quantity of antibody-rich plasma for the U.S. government supported COVID-19 expanded access program, accounting for roughly half of the supply used to treat 34,000 people." It was mostly due to such herculean humanitarian efforts that convalescent plasma became available in such a short time.

Whether convalescent plasma will have significant mortality benefits or not, only time will tell. However, preliminary studies (discussed more in Chapter Nine – Strategies to Combat COVID-19) do show benefit to patients if given early. That is what we experienced as physicians treating COVID-19 patients on the frontlines (although anecdotally). I am hopeful that patients who did and do benefit, no matter their background or religious persuasion, are eternally grateful to the local and extended Jewish community – you know, *those people.*

Bigotry and discrimination are not the sole province of religion. One of the multiple heads of this hydra also impacted the elderly community. Elderly people were dying more than the younger ones. This had two main deleterious results: one was the callous dismissal of the value of human life – the elderly human; and the second was the development of a misplaced sense of invincibility by the young, much to their own detriment. The second is not only one that will, over the years, continue to haunt certain young adults infected by the virus, but also in a diabolical twist of fate made them unaware or asymptomatic carriers of the virus that ended up infecting the elderly and frail.

Many hospitals saw their share of increased deaths among the elderly. Most of the deaths that occurred among the elderly belonged to the above 65 years age group, and typically patients who had additional medical problems and risk factors, such as diabetes mellitus, high blood pressure, obesity, chronic obstructive pulmonary disease and kidney failure. Many of them were in their 80s and 90s, while some were in their 70s. Many, for the most part, led productive lives, spending precious moments with their children, grandchildren, and great grandchildren, before they were infected by the deadly virus.

The disproportionate tragedy that COVID-19 has befallen on our elderly has exposed the moral bankruptcy that exists in our society even if it is in a small percentage. Even certain political leaders and so-called public servants like Tony Abbott, a former Prime Minister of Australia, reportedly suggested in a speech in the UK at the Policy Exchange think tank "that some elderly coronavirus patients could be left to die naturally." Abbott also purportedly said, "that governments were not thinking like health economists, trained to pose uncomfortable questions about a level of deaths we might have to live with." He continued by trying to place a monetary cost per life saved in Australia to a value of "$2 million per life saved – or $200,000 per year if they had only a 10 year life expectancy," which according to him would be "substantially beyond what governments are usually prepared to pay for lifesaving drugs."

Prepared to pay! First, governments and public servants are formed and elected to serve the people, all people – including the elderly. They better be prepared to serve and pay for lifesaving drugs or should just get out of the way! Second, it should not take $2 million to treat every COVID-19 patient – that is just an overinflated cost or cost due to mismanaged delivery of patient care with many people's hands in the money pot. Abbott's speech was at a Policy Exchange think tank! Another reason why healthcare should not be run by economists, but by clinical healthcare professionals who understand and can deliver efficient healthcare and patient care. More importantly, the clinical healthcare professionals, overwhelmingly, have their hearts and minds in the right place – both, morally and financially. As a result, they can effectively and efficiently provide uncompromised healthcare within the bounds of financial viability.

At times I can't help but wonder if administrators fell short on the types of assurances that many may have promised when soliciting the help of local community leaders, other physicians, and other hospital staff – we would not compromise on patient care – that is not what physicians and nurses do; we will try our best to provide all that is required and asked of us by the patient and the patient's family and respect their wishes and their lives; your community liaisons will be a life-line to the over-extended medical team and will be welcomed at our hospitals; of course, you'll be protected; money is not an issue when it comes to saving lives – that is not the American way.

Wonder how history will judge those administrators!

Dr. Rajesh Mohan

Chapter Eight

The Dogma of Bureaucracy

When people across the world think of hospitals, their minds immediately envision a maze of intersecting hallways that are uncreatively reproduced floor after floor in fairly non-descript buildings. Adding to this sterile environment are doctors in white coats and nurses in scrubs rushing from one patient to another in what appears to be a never-ending fight of comfort over pain, relief over anguish, and life over death.

The human drama at play in its more visceral form is too much for the senses of those outside healthcare to comprehend, and aside from periodic screams of pain that somehow manage to pierce their numbed senses, energies of most people remain focused on coping with this assault on their senses.

Deftly maneuvering within the same corridors, and in many instances, ensconced on different floors are the people who are managing, directing, and choreographing the entire flow – the Administrators. These are the people who determine the functioning of the entire hospital, from the number of ambulances arriving at the hospital's door, to how, by whom, and for how long the patients are to be treated.

It may surprise some to learn that when asked about the most respected profession in the world, doctors came in first. It may surprise even more to learn that lawyers came in second. Some believe this ranking stemmed more from need than anything else. Both professions seem to find their consumers (patients/clients) at their most vulnerable.

While the legal profession has seen certain changes over the decades, for the most part, the law firm structure has remained mostly the same. In contrast, the medical profession appears to have become increasingly bureaucratic, particularly in the U.S.

While the number of medical doctors has increased over the past few decades, it still falls short of the demonstrated need.

Of interest to note, however, is that the number of administrators has disproportionally increased by a multiple that, compared to the number of doctors they are meant to support, defies logic.

As per the Harvard Business Review, for every doctor there are 10 healthcare workers who are purely in administrative and management roles.

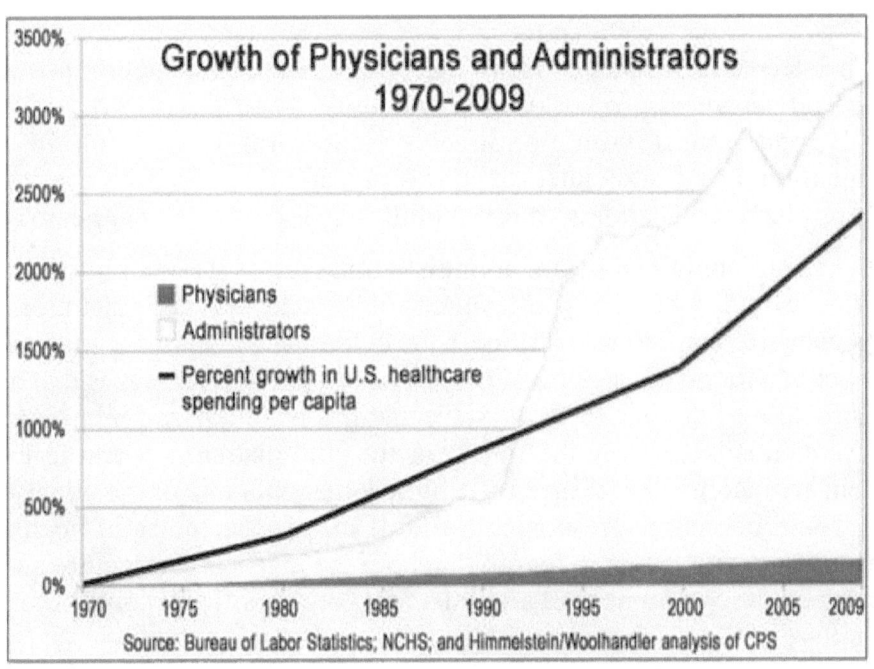

COVIDSLAYERS

Some might wonder that if the number of administrators has increased such, why is it that they are not as visible as they should be. This goes back to doctors being the most admired profession. Wouldn't you want to exploit the veneer of a busy and respected doctor to serve to insulate you from difficult questions and scrutiny?

This brings us to the next questions. Well, what do these administrators do that justify their exponential growth in numbers over the years, and their questionably high compensation? Based upon impressions from various economists and physicians, it appears that most of these administrators have no relevant clinical knowledge or experience and are paper-pushers, indulged in busy-work emanating from various governmental agencies, administering programs from state and federal governments, insurance companies, licensing and accreditation agencies, writing policies and protocols, enforce regulations and trying to tell doctors how to practice medicine.

The steep and sustained rise in the cost of healthcare superimposes the steep and sustained growth of administrators. Their busy work, which is mostly non-clinical with no direct patient care, in addition to their compensation and associated expenses, apparently would be the logical driver of increased padding of patient bills and increase in healthcare costs.

What is it about healthcare administration that while one physician can provide care for hundreds of patients in a year, 10 administrators per physician are required to administer the delivery of healthcare to the same number of patients? The apparent and possibly obvious answer is that either the structure of the healthcare system that has been devised by politicians and economists is highly inefficient or the administrators working in this system are incompetent. Since it is unlikely that only one or the other of the two would be entirely responsible for all the inefficiencies in healthcare administration, it stands to reason that both the inefficient structure and the incompetence of a number of administrators are significant contributors for the failure of healthcare administration.

Some of these paper-pushers apparently have incredulously boasted of writing numerous policies within 6 months and in the midst of this once-in-100-year pandemic. While I can only rely so much on the knowledge of my fellow physician and nursing colleagues as to whether the growth in numbers and compensation of the administrators are justified, what has become abundantly clear to many physicians and nurses over the past few decades, and highlighted over the COVID-19 pandemic, is that the role many administrators play is profoundly antithetical to the practice of medicine, and fell grossly short of expectations during the early stages of the COVID-19 pandemic, and continues to do so.

Of course, any hospital, much like any corporate entity, requires an administrative team. However, a one-to-one analogy cannot, and should not be drawn between a product manufacturing company and a hospital or any healthcare entity. For example, Apple® can decide to leave a certain enhancement or expense for their next version to maximize their return on investment (ROI) on the current one, but a hospital cannot (should not), for example, recycle or extend PPE use to save a nickel, especially if it is receiving federal funds to compensate for any perceived price gouging due to an anticipated reduced supply and high demand. Nor should obfuscation techniques gleaned from $5 business books bought off the pavement be used to provide patronizing answers to offset cost, especially when lives are at stake.

The modus operandi of healthcare administrators used to manage doctors, nurses, and other healthcare personnel in the U.S. healthcare system typically relies on peculiar strategies that deftly steer the focus away from actual patient–care to an emphasis on idiosyncratic, but endearing–sounding "quality" metrics that are often associated with financial incentives inversely related to patient care. These financially incentivized "quality" metrics are then relentlessly pursued while professing to provide "quality" healthcare to patients – many times at the cost of actual patient care.

The foregoing relies upon the ubiquitous acceptance of the term "quality" to serve as unquestionable acceptance and justification for any proposed change. We are often inundated with many a project, initiatives, endeavors often characterized as improving the "quality" of "service."

Thus, why would healthcare administrators leave the fertile field of medicine devoid of such changes, especially if such initiatives serve to secure their employment and compensation? Of course, adding improving the "quality of patient care," or improving the "quality of the patient experience," serve as euphemisms to the longevity of many healthcare administrators.

After all, what else has and continues to be the primary mandate of physicians and nurses.

Another questionable practice that exasperated many was one of deflection that many administrators had honed their skills on over decades by placing doctors and nurses at the forefront to insulate themselves. This practice seemed to be ubiquitously practiced across the country by many administrators echoing the sentiments of the partisan divide and blaming the federal government for not being prepared for the pandemic.

Really? You can apparently run hospitals, hospital systems and large healthcare organizations, tell doctors and nurses what to do and what "medical" protocols to follow (after you have stripped them to the bone with the only yardstick being the likelihood of a lawsuit), yet you need the federal government to prepare YOU for a medical emergency? Yes, we do need the federal government for national policy and guidelines as well as resources. However, we cannot and should not use the inactions and incompetence of others as excuses to hide our own shortcomings. Don't they teach contingency plans in whatever classes one takes to become an administrator? What other top 5 contingencies at a hospital and in healthcare can one consider that does not include an influx of patients with an unknown ailment or contagion? Especially, if Hollywood already thought of it nearly a decade ago!

As a consequence of the incompetence and disingenuous approach by administrator saturated healthcare agencies toward the pandemic, many physicians and physician leaders took it upon themselves to make sure that the increasing number of COVID-19 patients received the best possible care. In addition, they supported their nursing colleagues and pushed the administrators to make sure that adequate staffing for critical care nursing was made available, minimizing the exploitation of employed staff. Although the administrators should have ensured adequate staffing levels of respiratory therapists and other frontline healthcare personnel on their own, it was the physicians and physician leaders who pushed the administrators to wake them up from their slumber.

It was the constant drumbeat in the news media, multiple social media forum and local physician uprisings that forced administrators to take notice and acquiesce to providing some semblance of supply of PPE to all hospital employees, nursing staff and medical staff. If not for the physician leaders, the "difficult physicians" and, during this pandemic there were more than a few, penchant for making sure that all medical staff were adequately protected while working on the front lines which extended to all nurses and hospital staff, there could have been tragically more COVID-19 exposures and deaths among healthcare personnel.

Due to the vacuum created, not surprisingly because of the incapabilities of public and health officials, healthcare administrators, and the panic and confusion among healthcare administrators, physician leaders in many hospitals, for the most part, tried to steer day-to-day management that impacted patient care despite the handicap of not having financial or administrative powers. Influencing management would include not just what would pertain to direct patient care – it would extend to holding the hands of administrators, guiding, and even cajoling them into doing the right thing for the benefit of patients. Administrators were even cajoled into spending money to provide adequate number of critical care physicians 24x7 and not leave patient care in the hands of overworked and short-staffed physicians. The same extended to nurses, respiratory therapists, and other frontline healthcare personnel.

Physician leaders in many hospitals were even exposing their talents of handymen/women, construction, and plant operators. Their ideas led to methods where tubing and extension cords were connected to intravenous (IV) pumps which were then placed outside COVID-19 isolation rooms. This benefited nurses tremendously as now they could manage IV medications, IV fluids and IV pump alarms without going inside isolation rooms. This would decrease their exposure to COVID-19 as well as decrease the use of rationed PPE. In addition, they could administer medications in a more timely manner without having to put on and take off PPE in every instance. Similar ideas by physician leaders led to configuring of extensions for ventilators which were then modified leading to the monitors being placed outside isolation rooms of COVID-19 patients who were intubated. Respiratory therapists and physicians, including intensivists, who may have to adjust parameters of ventilators of multiple such patients' multiple times a day, would as a result have decreased exposure time to COVID-19. This would decrease their exposure and risk of infection by airborne transmission from such patients. This would also decrease the use of rationed PPE.

Physician leaders in hospitals also stepped in to fill in the roles of contractors. Many hospitals had setup triage tents outside ERs with the goal to move COVID-19 patients quickly and efficiently, thereby avoiding clogging up the ER. COVID-19 patients were recommended to be in admitted to negative pressure isolation rooms. Not surprisingly, according to many physicians and nurses a sense of urgency was lacking in the bureaucratic and the contractor mindsets – even during this pandemic. Physician leaders at various sites would guide and even physically be present to make sure tasks were completed in time. It appears that minds, belief systems and dogmatic thinking of many in the bureaucracy gives them reassurance in a false sense of competence that they become accustomed to in their glacial pace of activity and decision making. Their dogmatic thinking takes a lot of "pushing" to not only make them recognize the obvious but also bring them up to the speed that is required to function efficiently in a dynamic environment.

COVID-19 has a wide-ranging destructive impact on the human body. As sicker patients were admitted to critical care units with progressive complications including kidney failure, it was only a matter of time that limits were going to be reached in terms of dialysis capabilities in hospitals. Hospitals would require more dialysis machines, more dialysis nurses and dialysis technicians. Did the administrators have a clue about this? Did they start counting the cost of providing this essential care? Physician leaders would again push them to do the right thing for patients.

Patients were still being told by public officials as well as health administrators that they should stay home if they had mild and moderate symptoms and seek hospital care only when they were "really" sick and had severe symptoms. As a result, more patients came to the hospital in late stages when they required critical care, intubations, and ventilators. In anticipation of this surge, hospitals were required to ramp up their critical care bed capacity with negative pressure capability. At the insistence of and pressure from physician leaders in various hospitals, bureaucrats and contractors again were reluctantly dragged out of their entrenched comfort zones. It was essential for the non-clinical bureaucracy, financial administrators, and contractors to rise out of their state of inertia to efficiently deliver in a dynamic environment. It was necessary to do so, to make sure that appropriate infrastructure was available for the clinical staff so that they could then provide the best possible care to patients.

With more COVID-19 patients came more PPE usage – especially in the COVID cohorted ICU patient rooms. Staff, especially intensivists, nurses and nurses' aides who were there for long hours in close proximity of COVID-19 patients in those units had to be fully protected. Utilization of PPE, N95 masks and bunny suits (disposable protective coverall safety suit) would come into question. As per nurses and physicians in hospitals, there was a "push" from administrators to use a poncho (with no back cover and hood) as it was cheaper than the bunny suit. Physicians, physician leaders and nurses knew that a poncho would be inadequate protection. Nurses and other employees would reach out to physicians for support as they were afraid of repercussions.

It was obvious to the frontline warriors in hospitals, that no amount of cost of a bunny suit (about $5 to $25 depending upon the company) was worth more than a human life – especially those of frontline healthcare personnel who were already putting their lives on the line to care for patients. Most knew that patients could transmit a potentially mortal infection to healthcare personnel which could then spread to their families as well. By now, with increasing media attention and vocal nurses and physicians at many hospitals, healthcare personnel at many hospitals knew that if administrators were going to ask them to manage patient care during a pandemic with dollars and cents in their minds, well then – it was their cost of doing business.

COVIDSLAYERS

Physicians and physician leaders at hospitals would come to the rescue again!

Where were all the healthcare administrators during all this? – Oh, in their offices or "working from home."

Was there even a need for them – so many of them?

Is there any need for them – so many of them?

Dr. Rajesh Mohan

COVIDSLAYERS

Chapter Nine

The Inhumane Visitors Policy

Was the draconian visitor policy really necessary?

As patients with COVID started getting admitted to hospitals, the fear that these patients would spread the infection started getting hold. Who could these patients transmit the infection to?

There were only two sets of people who could possibly get infected from these COVID-19 patients. The *first* group of people would be healthcare personnel – doctors, nurses, respiratory therapists, phlebotomists, nurses' aides, and any other healthcare personnel who would come in their contact while taking care of them in the hospital. The *second* group of people would be the family and friends who may visit a patient when the patient is admitted and being treated in the hospital. For the most part, a loved one – wife, husband, son, or daughter – who wanted to visit the patient may have already been exposed to the patient prior to the patient coming to the hospital.

Short sightedly and reflexively, agencies and hospitals decided that they would severely constrain visitation of patients when admitted to hospitals. As a result, visitations for the most part would be restricted to extenuating circumstances such as if admitted patients were on hospice or end of life. Baby monitors, FaceTime and iPads for communications among patients and family members were being used. They served as valuable adjuncts and were better than nothing at all. However, the invaluable feeling of a touch by a loved one could not have been substituted in any way.

In most, if not all hospitals, visitors were screened at the hospital entrance. If the visitors failed screening – which was if they had any fever or symptoms or had a travel history to one of the states identified by the NJDOH within 14 days, then they were not allowed to visit their loved ones.

Think about this for a second and picture the following potential scenario.

An admitted patient in a hospital is at end of life and therefore about to die. The loved ones – a daughter, a son, a husband or a wife are not allowed to visit the patient who lay on his or her deathbed because the family member(s) may have had a fever or had a travel history to one of the listed areas. What harm, if any, would the family member cause to a dying loved one? And, if the concerns were that the family member would infect a hospital staff member, then what was the hinderance in making sure that the visiting family member was covered with appropriate PPE? And, if the hospital was rationing PPE (which should not be 9 months into the pandemic) and therefore was unable to provide PPE to a family member, and if the family member was able to procure their own PPE, then there should have been no reason for any barriers to visitation that was structured, controlled and humane. In addition, there was no reason for any hospital employee to be in the close proximity of the family member coming to visit a dying loved one. It defies commonsense!

Many hospitals had implemented stringent visitor policies. In scenarios where a patient was COVID-19 positive and was on mechanical ventilation, and not at end of life, the family members were offered the use of an iPad or FaceTime to see their loved one. If the patient was COVID-19 positive or under investigation for COVID-19 but not on a ventilator, visitation was still restricted with an alternative of an iPad or FaceTime communication being the only option. Even if patients tested negative for COVID-19 and were admitted to a hospital, initially all visitation was restricted – they were later on, allowed one visitor per day for a few minutes.

All these restrictions were apparently put in place in hospitals, so that the one or two immediate family members – the wife, the husband, the daughter, or the son does not carry the infection from the patient to the community or potentially infect hospital staff. The underlying and main reason for such restrictions in place would again unmistakably lead to what was cited as a shortage of N95 masks and other PPE. If healthcare personnel were unable to be provided with adequate N95 masks and PPE, then how could the visitors be provided with the same while visiting their loved ones – it was reasoned. And, if a loved one did not wear N95 masks and appropriate PPE while visiting, then they were at risk of not only contracting COVID-19 but also propagating the infection to others in the community and the hospital staff. Shortage and rationing of N95 masks and PPE were obvious and many times valid reasons to deny visitation to loved ones.

What was the fault of the helpless patient and the distraught and equally helpless loved one? The critical role that the loved ones of a patient have in the successful treatment of any patient was forgotten and discarded.

Again, "Guidelines and policies" emanating from the DOH, the state government, or hospital systems were made to justify such restrictions. These included verbiage like "extenuating circumstances" which were up for interpretation and would cause more confusion. It became apparent that unclear language and caveats were placed intentionally or unintentionally in such "guidelines and policies" which were then being used to deny visitation coupled with plausible deniability in cases of dispute. Examples such as end of life and hospice were given for "extenuating circumstances" with the door left a little open with phrases such as "not limited to" such circumstances.

This was (is) the scenario in all hospitals throughout New York, New Jersey, and the country. Minds had been made. Patients in isolation and solitary confinement was going to be the norm. Tragically, many patients who would recover from these harrowing experiences would forever be scarred with a fear of the hospital leaving an indelible mark on their psyche.

What was/is the need to play such games if patient and family well-being are the primary and sole aim of healthcare?

Patient care, of which family support is an integral component, should be the sole aim of healthcare – pandemic or no pandemic!

Patients were dying in isolation, alone. Family members were having a difficult time accepting the circumstances and were distraught and helpless. They were having a difficult time achieving a reasonable sense of closure with an emotional trauma that would linger for an unknown period of time.

In addition, nurses and doctors who were at bedside would not only witness the last precious moments of patients on behalf of families, but also functioned as a substitute of loved ones, passing along last messages to the best of their abilities.

Doctors and nurses are always acutely aware that the "fear of dying alone is nearly universal." They "go to great lengths to give patients just a little more time for family members to arrive and say their goodbyes." What was considered compassionate although challenging but always an earnest promise that doctors and nurses would try to keep – "We'll do everything we can to keep him alive until you get here," changed to, "Because of hospital policy, we cannot allow visitors at this time." In addition to the heroic work that they were immersed in on the frontlines, supporting this cop out was not what the healthcare personnel had expected to be their roles. This would undoubtedly result in a significant emotional toll and in many cases guilt that they would carry thereafter.

Visitations were restricted to such an extent that when an ambulance was called to transport a family member to a hospital, many family members thought and felt as if that would be the last time they would be seeing their loved one.

Many hospitals, including hospitals such as Brigham and Women's were reported to have "barred visitors, even for patients at the end of their lives, out of concern that visitors could help the new coronavirus spread throughout the hospital." Patients were left "to suffer through their illness in a medical version of solitary confinement," stated Dr. Daniela J. Lamas, a critical care doctor, according to the New York Times dated March 24, 2020. Patients would die "in separate sterile hospital rooms, far from anyone who loves them," she continued in the New York Times. Across hospitals, loved ones were being told to say their last goodbyes at the time of admission to hospitals. As stated in the same opinion piece, many times husbands and wives or other family members who were admitted to hospitals, died alone. In the days and weeks to come, these tragic scenarios were going to be repeated too many times in hospitals across the country.

Tragically, even those patients who did recover from COVID would carry with them the scarred experience resulting from solitary confinement and the banishment of family support during a time when it was most crucial.

As per a local community leader and a Rabbi, a Jewish prayer – Mi Sheberach – for those who are sick was being frequently offered even while patients were in the process of being stretchered into ambulances to be taken to a nearby hospital. This was being done as a result of the fear that it may be the last time that the patient would be seen.

Mostly as a cop-out, but in the minds of middle men and people who had minimal idea of patient care if any, this was an opportunity to substitute human touch with technology, and at the same time convert this tragedy to a money making opportunity. The word "technology" is fashionably thrown around and in many instances, gratuitously touted as a panacea for all challenges in healthcare. This occurs even when recommended technologies are themselves still in their infancy. Unbeknownst to many, physicians, and medicine, in general, have been leaders in technological innovation and adaptation with a maturity level that is far advanced, and which exceeds many other industries including the nascent information technology industry.

How could the last picture of a dying patient with tubes sticking out of the mouth and nose and secretions including blood and bile pouring out, give comfort or provide any level of solace or closure to a loved one? How could the tender touch and feelings of meeting hands and lips be replaced by the touch of an iPad screen?

Many such "technological miracles" have been pushed into healthcare blindly and hurriedly. This has been done without much regard nor accountability for the well-being or with a proven benefit for the patient. They can be used at best as an adjunct to the human touch of medicine but certainly not at the tremendous cost of replacing it.

Upstart unproven technologies which are mostly associated with mediocrity have no place in an advanced field of science such as medicine where human touch is essential and human lives are at stake. Many underdeveloped technologies with limited scope have, for the most part, come and gone or have not risen from their nascent stages while trying their best to relegate humanity. These suboptimal technologies do make a lot of money for a lot of people–even if it is a quick buck mostly at the expense of fellow human beings and unnecessary deviation from human care.

Only smart technologies, when developed and used in medicine, keeping the humanity of medicine as their primary objective rather than its relegation, have been successful.

It was abhorrent to comprehend that the incompetence to secure adequate PPE was used to support – and many times used as an excuse for – the inhumane visitation restrictions.

An informed humanitarian approach would have seen to the timely production and procurement of PPE, in addition to manufacturing more COVID-19 tests, and aggressively explored where technology would have and can make not only the most significant but probably the easiest impact towards vanquishing this pandemic.

But, for these "technology pushers," the ROI for mass production and procurement of PPE is probably not good enough. If they would have made PPE in large numbers, the cost of PPE would have gone lower and down to what was prior to the pandemic. N95 masks would cost about 58 cents or less, instead of $7 dollars, and not only healthcare personnel, but the general public could afford and wear them without spending significantly more money. This would obviously have had helped in the mitigation and containment of the COVID-19 pandemic.

Alas, ROI is more important than humanity!

Is the existence of our healthcare system for the benefit of patients? Or is our healthcare system supposed to be an industry where "cost" is the primary motivator and everything else, including patient care, is secondary and open to compromise and degradation – including life.

COVIDSLAYERS

Visitation policies in many hospitals would remain restricted with no significant changes even until 8 months after the initial surge had subsided. The opinion piece of Dr. Lamas on March 24, 2020 in the New York Times came and went. Numerous nurses and physicians have since expressed their anguish and pain about watching patients die alone with no loved one at the bedside. Many nurses and doctors have placed themselves on a daily basis as substitutes of family members, at the bedside of lonely and scared patients, in attempts to provide solace and reassurance. Often enough, they are the only ones at the bedside during the last few moments of a dying patient's life on planet Earth.

These brave souls try to do the best that they can in circumstances that they never envisioned to be in. They volunteer to place themselves in these agonizing conditions even at their own personal peril, so as to try to provide the human touch that a family member would have and could have willingly provided.

Patients and patient families have been pleading throughout this pandemic for a humane visitor policy. Family members have been more than willing to comply with full PPE requirements and even being escorted to and from their sick loved ones. Some hospitals have recognized the anguish of patients and family members and are providing requisite PPE, staff, and resources to facilitate limited visitation. Many hospitals are still counting dollars and cents due to the expense associated with relaxing their visitor policies. Hiding behind a false premise of "potential" infection to the hospital staff, visitor policies at many hospitals still remain draconian.

There is no reason that visitors cannot be allowed for patients who are sick and admitted to hospitals – COVID or non-COVID – as there is minimal risk, if any, to hospital staff and the visitors, as long as all are provided and wear appropriate PPE.

Even if the easiest and "ideal" solution (sans ulterior pecuniary objectives) is to quarantine patients with zero visitation rights, a balance ought to be sought to mitigate projected risks, e.g., by providing PPE, yet allowing visitations. If the same heartless logic and thought process in the pursuit of an "ideal" solution were to be extended outside the venerable halls of hospitals, we would ALL be under lockdown.

Dr. Rajesh Mohan

Have we all become so anesthetized to the sufferings of patients that while we condemn the "draconian" lockdown measures by certain Asian countries, we condone their application to our own sick, just as long as no one suggests that we be under a similar lockdown and are prevented from seeing anyone outside our households? I would like to think not. But it does make it an easier pill to swallow if guised as a new "protocol" sponsored and promoted by healthcare administrators across the nation, doesn't it?

Do hospitals have draconian visitor policies so that they can discourage COVID-19 patients from coming to their hospitals? Do they want to discourage or limit COVID-19 patients from coming to their hospital so that they can continue "business as usual" and keep other money-making services open? Do they want to save a few bucks that would be spent on PPE, at the expense of emotional and mental well-being of patients whose care they are responsible for?

Anti-patient draconian policies have no place in healthcare. Such healthcare entities would have failed their patients and the communities that they are supposed to serve. They would have failed in their mission to serve, which is the mandate of every healthcare entity.

Sooner or later, patients and communities will realize that such hospitals were not there by their side at the time when they needed them the most.

Why would patients go to such hospitals for their non-COVID needs?

Facilitation of patient visits by their loved ones is not only good for patient recovery and their mental and emotional well-being, but the right and humane thing to do.

And, if nothing else, it is the cost of doing business.

Chapter Ten

Strategies to Combat COVID-19

Almost every day since March 14, 2020, mostly in the evenings, I would call Dr. Kumar to find out how he was doing.

Dr. Kumar continued to have high fever almost every day for about 10-12 days since his initial diagnosis of COVID-19. He was checking his temperature at least a couple of times a day. He was also checking his oxygen saturation regularly. He felt very weak, but in spite of multiple suggestions to come to the hospital, he chose not to, as he had confidence that he could manage his condition at home. From day one, he had already started taking hydroxychloroquine, Vitamin C, Vitamin D, Zinc, and azithromycin. He was taking acetaminophen round the clock to control his fever and was replenishing himself with liquids and electrolytes.

In addition to the medications, fluids and electrolytes, Dr. Kumar was regularly laying on his stomach for hours, especially when his oxygen level would drop (below mid 90s). This laying on his stomach would increase his oxygen levels and make his breathing better for the next few hours, thus preventing the need to require assistance in breathing, thereby, reducing the odds of having to be rushed to the hospital.

It had been shown that turning onto their stomachs patients who were intubated with advanced involvement of the lung in a condition called acute respiratory distress syndrome (ARDS) had better outcomes. When COVID-19 patients with pneumonia deteriorated and required intubation and a ventilator, their pneumonia worsened and they usually, progressively deteriorated into the condition called ARDS. Without going into scientific minutiae, the thought process was to improve aeration of the lungs, especially the areas affected by COVID-19 and prevent worsening of breathing requiring intubation and a ventilator with the potential of progression to ARDS.

Dr. Kumar, despite his sickness, increased his voraciousness about learning all there was to learn about COVID-19. Although he came close to being sick enough to need hospitalization a few times, he was fortunately able to take care of himself at home without needing to rush to the ED. Starting the day of his initial diagnosis, Dr. Kumar and I used to have a conversation almost every day for the next 3 weeks. Although the main purpose of my calls was to make sure that he was doing well, he soon became one of the sources who I could rely upon to get an up-to-date progress in the management strategies being tried, practiced and published on a daily basis. Due to lingering effects of COVID-19, Dr. Kumar was able to join the fight against COVID-19 in about 3 weeks – April 3, 2020, instead of the 14 days that was initially anticipated.

Soon thereafter, there were other physicians who became sick with COVID-19, with whom I would also converse with on a regular basis. All of them were fortunate to win their fights against COVID-19 and eventually return to battle at their hospitals or medical practices.

Discussing with these physicians on a daily basis, particularly Dr. Kumar, I practically had my own personal COVID-19 journal club and review meetings, assessing management strategies that they were employing themselves in their own personal fights against this dreaded virus, and those that they were keeping up to date with and following in real-time.

COVIDSLAYERS

By the time Dr. Kumar returned from his own personal battle with COVID-19, we in the hospital were right in the midst of a full-scale war with COVID-19. His personal experiences with COVID-19, which included managing the critical days prior to, during, and after the notorious hyper-inflammatory response of the body to the virus commonly known as the cytokine storm, and eventually winning his personal battle against COVID-19, was a major morale booster to the hospital staff.

There were also frequent communications and exchange of ideas, experiences, and treatment strategies among physicians. This occurred not only among physicians taking care of patients within the hospital and the local community but also crossed state and international borders. Experiences of Individual physicians as well as groups of physicians personally treating COVID-19 patients on the frontlines (not state or government reported experiences which were not entirely reliable) shared their experiences in real-time, either by direct contact or on secure apolitical physician groups on social media. Most treatment modalities were experimental and off-label.

Most physicians, by nature and their training, are not ones to throw in their towels and surrender, especially when they are placed in situations of life and death where they are asked and expected to bring out their best. Providing only supportive care and hoping for the best is not what most physicians signed up for nor would that have measured up to their calling while facing a once-in-a-100–years pandemic and once in a lifetime medical challenge of epic proportions. Anyone could provide supportive care and hope for the best. Physicians have been educated and trained to stretch boundaries and provide the best possible care that they can humanly provide.

The critical thinking and creative thinking of physicians went into top gear and reached unprecedented heights during this pandemic. Dogma of socialist "treatment protocols" and "order sets" – impediments to creative and critical thinking were left by the wayside. One of the basic principles in medicine that physicians' practice by is – first, do no harm. As long as plausible management strategies were safe, and did not cause harm to patients, they were considered.

Dr. Rajesh Mohan

Many have said that despite the reckless abandon with which the virus has spread and infected people in the US, it is a testament to the advanced knowledge, training, expertise and critical thinking capabilities of physicians which has resulted in their innovative COVID-19 management strategies that resulted in fewer people dying than would have otherwise.

In the absence of a cure or a vaccine for COVID-19, there has been no magic bullet or one particular medication that has shown to successfully combat this potentially deadly virus. It has been usually a combination of treatments strategies based upon a patient's condition which has helped. It is a tribute to the medical community that they have improvised whatever is available and modulated those into management strategies and treatment cocktails which have been used in an amorphous manner dependent upon individual patient scenarios.

Many of them like Vitamin C, Zinc, and Vitamin D are mostly innocuous. They are available as over-the-counter supplements and are not known to cause patient harm or death even in slightly higher than usual doses when used for a short period of time.

Laying patients on their stomach (proning), including those who were on a ventilator, as long as they were being observed and monitored in a controlled environment, was similarly harmless to a patient.

In the early days of the pandemic, based upon scientific data available at the time and with the input of other physicians who were managing COVID-19 patients, I developed a *COVID-19 Management Protocol* giving physicians liberty to use their own clinical judgment to modify strategies that they may deem appropriate for the benefit of their patients. It goes without saying that for every management modality, the principle of *first, do no harm* is always expected to be in the forefront of physicians' minds. This protocol was similar to those in many other hospitals throughout the state and the country, which is a testament to the high degree of exchange of scientific and medical knowledge as well as communication among physicians in the same hospital, across state lines and among different specialties of medicine.

COVIDSLAYERS

The protocol started with, as usual, an initial assessment of a patient in the emergency department. After the initial assessment, certain lab tests and a test for COVID-19 were obtained.

As in most hospitals, laboratory assessment at the time of admission included blood work which included tests like complete blood count (CBC), comprehensive metabolic panel (CMP), Fibrinogen, Troponin, lactic acid, c- reactive protein (CRP) (Non-Cardiac), lactate dehydrogenase (LDH), Ferritin, Magnesium, Phosphorus, D-dimer, procalcitonin and prothrombin time/ international normalized ration/activated partial thromboplastin time (PT/INR/aPTT). In COVID-19 confirmed patients and as per treating physicians, laboratory tests after admission on a daily basis mostly included CMP, CBC, Magnesium, Phosphorus, D-dimer, PT/INR/aPTT, Ferritin and CRP (Non-Cardiac).

In the early days. all COVID-19 patients, for the most part and as per treating physicians, received hydroxychloroquine for up to 4-10 days, Zinc, Vitamin C, Vitamin D3, Thiamine and Melatonin. If treating physicians suspected concomitant infection such as pneumonia, then broad-spectrum antibiotics were added. Steroids, mostly IV steroids, were given especially in patients who had decreased oxygen levels and had difficulty breathing requiring oxygen. Anticoagulation (blood thinners) with dose based upon D-dimer levels were also given to patients. Patients were also treated with bronchodilators (medicines that widen the airways) such as albuterol plus ipratropium or albuterol. Antacids such as famotidine were prescribed as well. Oxygen at high-flow rates were given to patients who had difficulty breathing unless they decompensated and required intubation and being placed on a ventilator. Some patients, based upon physician assessment, were also given Tocilizumab, an Interleukin-6 antagonist which has been touted to have action against the dreaded cytokine storm. What also helped in many cases was laying patients on their stomach (proning) when patients were on a medical floor and not intubated as well as when patients were in critical care unit and intubated on a mechanical ventilator.

Hydroxychloroquine as a treatment has been extensively politicized. It is true that it has not been proven to have any benefit in the treatment of COVID-19 patients, as has been touted to by one extreme of the political spectrum. It is also true that it is not a dangerous drug causing rampant death due to cardiac arrhythmias as has been sensationalized by the other extreme end of the political spectrum.

The NIH, after its fourth interim analysis decided to stop "a clinical trial being to evaluate the safety and effectiveness of hydroxychloroquine for the treatment of adults hospitalized with coronavirus disease 2019 (COVID-19)." The data and safety monitoring board (DSMB) "determined that while there was no harm, the study drug was very unlikely to be beneficial to hospitalized patients with COVID-19." The NIH advisory stated that "Study shows treatment does no harm, but provides no benefit."

As per the American College of Cardiology (ACC) in an article published on March 29, 2020, "Chloroquine and its more contemporary derivative hydroxychloroquine, have remained in clinical use for more than half-century as an effective therapy for treatment of some malarias, lupus, and rheumatoid arthritis. Data shows inhibition of iKr (iKr – inward rectifier potassium channel present in heart cells) and resultant mild QT (measurement between the Q and T wave in an electrocardiogram) prolongation associated with both agents. Despite these suggestive findings, several hundred million courses of chloroquine have been used worldwide making it one of the most widely used drugs in history, without reports of arrhythmic death under World Health Organization surveillance."

The same ACC article goes onto absolve even azithromycin and its combination with chloroquine by stating that, "Azithromycin, a frequently used macrolide antibiotic lacks strong pharmacodynamic evidence of iKr inhibition. Epidemiologic studies have estimated an excess of 47 cardiovascular deaths which are presumed arrhythmic per 1 million completed courses, although recent studies suggest this may be overestimated." It also states that, "there is limited data evaluating the safety of combination therapy, however in vivo studies have shown no synergistic arrhythmic effects of azithromycin with or without chloroquine."

In fact, numerous patients with lupus and rheumatoid arthritis have taken and continue to take hydroxychloroquine for months and years with many of them not even getting an electrocardiogram recorded. None of them undergo continuous, ongoing heart monitoring looking for any arrhythmias, nor is it recommended. They tolerate the medicine well with no reported cardiac deaths related to arrhythmias due to hydroxychloroquine. In contrast, for patients with COVID-19 in whom hydroxychloroquine was being considered as an option for treatment, the drug was mostly being given only for a maximum of 10 days.

In short, hydroxychloroquine is a safe drug especially when used for a short duration but has no proven benefit for the treatment of COVID-19.

The other members of the treatment protocol – Zinc, Vitamin C, Vitamin D3, Thiamine and Melatonin – have an excellent safety profile and are not known to cause any known significant harm, especially when taken for a short duration. They are used based upon the rationale that they help the immune system and may have significant anti-inflammatory and anti-viral activity at high doses.

Tocilizumab has been part of several trials with mixed results. However, preliminary results from the Evaluating Minority Patients with Actemra (EMPACTA) trial have shown that COVID-19 "hospitalized patients who received tocilizumab were 44% less likely to progress to mechanical ventilation or death compared with patients who received placebo plus standard of care."

Steroids (dexamethasone) have now been shown to decrease deaths when given to patients that are hospitalized with COVID-19 as per the Randomized Evaluation of COVID-19 Therapy (RECOVERY) trial. Many physicians in hospitals across the U.S. had been seeing benefits of steroid use and had started using them prior to the results of this trial. This was apparently based upon clinical experiences and observation of excess inflammation seen in COVID-19 patients especially those with a severe manifestation of the disease.

Blood thinners (anticoagulation) have also been shown to be beneficial in patients with COVID-19 who meet criteria.

Since the early days of the COVID-19 pandemic, other treatment modalities have been added to the armamentarium to fight the disease. One of them is Remdesivir—an anti-viral drug, which shortened "the time to recovery in adults hospitalized with COVID-19 and evidence of lower respiratory tract infection."

Convalescent plasma, for which preliminary data suggested but not confirmed, benefits patients with COVID-19 who are not intubated and those with less than a week of symptoms. It is approved for use under an Emergency Use Authorization (EUA) for the treatment of hospitalized patients with COVID-19.

There are numerous medications, therapeutics, and vaccines that the innovative scientific community is in a feverish race to develop to combat this deadly pandemic. These are in various stages of development and trials – some of them may not be successful, but hopefully more will show a significant benefit in combating COVID-19.

If all goes well, then frontrunners such as Moderna, Pfizer and BioNTech, and possibly AstraZeneca, may be able to make and distribute the vaccine by the end of 2020 or early 2021 to a pre-determined select group of people in the U.S. Some of the other companies like Sanofi, GlaxoSmithKline, and Merck may have their vaccines ready by the spring or summer of 2021.

Even if a cure or vaccine is developed, there will be a considerable amount of time before it would be easily available to all Americans. Even when we do have a cure or a vaccine, we may still need to adapt and follow certain preventive measures in order to contain the spread of this very contagious and deadly virus.

We as individuals and as a society at large cannot just stand by idly until treatments and/or vaccines that show proven effectiveness in curing the disease or vanquishing the virus are widely and easily available for the common man.

Too many people have died preventable deaths. It is a shame to our intelligence and our collective conscience that we as humans have even allowed this virus to bring us to our knees.

COVIDSLAYERS

We cannot allow the virus to be the harbinger of death to an increasing number of humans.

It is a war between the intellect and conscience of humankind versus the agility and random killing that is being perpetrated by the virus.

Catch the Virus and Nip It in the Bud

Many would say it is too late.

After so many deaths and so much havoc created by the virus, it would be the expected refrain flowing from conventional wisdom. But how long are we supposed to play defense and hide from the virus – which is invisible? Have we stooped down to such low levels of helplessness that our innovative and resourceful ingenuity has been so blunted that we do not even have the courage to believe in our own God gifted abilities? I do not believe so! There are more than enough innumerable valiant warriors among us that we as humans could never accept capitulation, ever.

With this as the basic premise, how do we then embark on a mission to catch the virus and nip it in the bud? How do we slay the virus? The good news is that we have done it before. We have beat back and ended infections with varying levels of success depending upon how persistent and innovative we have intended to be. We have been fighting infections – viruses, bacteria, and other organisms of various kinds since a long time and have been mostly successful.

Without going into a history lesson, many infectious diseases (and infectious agents associated with them) have significantly been deemed eradicated, cured, made inconsequential or are manageable. These include Hepatitis C, Influenza, Rabies, Leprosy, Typhoid Fever, Bubonic and Pneumonic Plagues, Cholera, Ebola, Middle East respiratory syndrome (MERS), Hantavirus, Anthrax, Pertussis, Meningitis–viral and bacterial, Syphilis, severe acute respiratory syndrome (SARS), Measles, Zika, Rabbit fever, Rotavirus, Bird flu, and, Tuberculosis to mention some.

So how do we catch and kill the new infectious agent – a virus called the severe acute respiratory syndrome coronavirus 2 (SARS-CoV-2)? To do so, there are some methods that are proven best practices that apply universally for the prevention of most infections but particularly to the spread of the disease COVID-19 caused by the SARS-CoV-2 virus.

Number one is – *Respect personal and universal hygiene and practice it unselfishly – wear a mask* – if we all do so, then we will organically respect the hygiene of others which will be the only way how any one of us will be able to practice hygiene for ourselves seamlessly and effectively. Practicing hygiene that is only selfishly limited to oneself makes it frequently limited to only one's own benefit and quite often at the expense of others. As a result, although the intention is to practice hygiene for oneself, most efforts could be negated by another person who may also have the same mindset and could also work selfishly only for his or her own personal hygiene disregarding and thereby negatively impacting the hygiene of others.

An example is our roads and highways. If people only thought about keeping their own cars clean, they would then throw trash out of their car windows while driving, resulting in littering of trash on our roads and highways. Most people do not throw trash outside their cars to keep their own cars clean, which they could (although fined if caught), resulting in clean roads. It is the same concept. Until we vanquish COVID-19, all of us should wear a mask if we are not alone, so that if anyone of us who could be carrying the virus (asymptomatic about 40%, asymptomatic or mild about 80%, symptomatic are about 15% with a high viral load) would not infect another person. This would be the same for someone else who could be carrying the virus and have the same or higher risk of infecting you if that person did not wear a mask negating all your efforts to prevent yourself from getting infected.

A study in the Journal of the American Medical Association showed "that a cough can spread droplets 13 to 16 feet and a sneeze can spread droplets up to 26 feet away." Therefore, anyone can get infected if another person coughs or sneezes while not wearing a mask and is 13 to 26 feet away. This can happen to anyone, anywhere without even knowing that someone has transmitted the infection. Therefore, as the Bible says – *"do unto others as you would have them do unto you"* – which for COVID-19 implies that if you do not infect others, then you would not get infected by another.

All should wear a mask until we vanquish COVID-19 together.

Number two is – *Wash Your Hands Often or use a hand sanitizer* – this may seem obvious, but not surprisingly, is not practiced as commonly as we all believe that it should. Many men, especially, have practiced and would be familiar with the *no touch technique* when they go to the bathroom to urinate so as to be able to justify their wrong practice to not wash their hands. In restaurants, as per the CDC, "only 1in 4 workers washed their hands after preparing raw animal products or handling dirt equipment, and only1 in 10 workers washed their hands after touching their face or body." Even among healthcare personnel, there have been studies that "show that some healthcare providers practice hand hygiene less than half of the times they should." It is essential that we wash hands after using the toilet, before eating, after coughing and sneezing, before and after preparing food, and after touching or handling objects that may have come across many other individuals.

Remember, COVID-19 can stay alive on plastic for about 72 hours. Therefore, wash your hands with soap and water for at least 20 seconds. It is interesting to note that a virus that has caused so much havoc in the lives of so many can be killed by soap if it is present on an external surface.

Number three is – *Cough or Sneeze into a tissue, napkin, handkerchief or into your elbow instead of your hands* – the CDC and the WHO have finally acquiesced to accepting that SARS-CoV-2 (the virus that causes COVID-19) can be spread via airborne transmission in addition to contact and droplet transmission. This can occur in enclosed spaces especially without adequate ventilation and air circulation, after exertional activities such as shouting, singing, and exercising even after the person carrying the virus has left the area. The virus in such an area could then be hanging around in the air, or droplets may have been deposited on surfaces. A person who would walk into such areas shortly thereafter and inhale the same virus infested air or touch the contaminated surface could then get infected. If there is adequate air circulation or such activities are carried out in open air environments, the risk of getting infected is significantly less.

A study showed that "the odds that a primary case transmitted COVID-19 in a closed environment was 18.7 times greater compared to an open-air environment." This would also follow commonsense which would suggest that the virus from any infected person in the air would be dispersed more and easier in an open-air environment with the virus clusters in droplets breaking up into small or individual numbers. This would make it less likely for the virus to "become concentrated in one area in the air and then inhaled by another person, which can result in infection."

As a result, when people are outdoors, it is less likely that they would "breathe in enough of the respiratory droplets containing the virus that causes COVID-19 to become infected." Even if a few virus particles are inhaled, the immune defenses of most people are capable of defeating the virus when it is in small numbers.

However, the risk even outdoors is not insignificant if people are in close proximity and without masks. In addition to being outdoors, if there is physical distancing of more than 6 feet and if everyone is wearing a mask, the risk then drops significantly.

Number four is – *practice physical distancing of at least 6 feet* – to prevent getting infected by droplets carrying the COVID-19 virus that may be released from another person while speaking.

Do not be socially distant, be physically distant.

Researchers at the University of Pennsylvania and the National Institute of Diabetes and Digestive and Kidney Diseases have shown that "2,600 small droplets were produced per second while talking." They also found that "speaking louder could generate larger droplets, as well as greater quantities of them…….and, estimated that a single minute of loud speaking could generate at least 1,000 virus-containing droplets." The rationale used is that most and especially large COVID-19 causing virus laden droplets would apparently drop within 6 feet and therefore not be inhaled. However, recent studies have shown that 6 feet may not be enough and farther the distance, the lesser the risk of getting infected.

COVIDSLAYERS

In addition, the longer you stay within 6 feet, the more virus you could be inhaling.

The amount of the SARS-CoV-2 virus necessary to make a person sick with COVID-19 is so far unknown. However, due to the ease of infection and rapid spread of the disease, the amount of virus required to cause the infection (infectious dose) is thought to be low.

Therefore, wearing a mask in combination with physical distancing would enhance protection and decrease the probability of getting infected. Masks of all variations must be mainly disposable and easily affordable and available – similar or even more than what they were before the pandemic. In addition, mask use strategies in different scenarios, based on risks, have been devised which are easy to follow for all Americans and should be put into practice. As a result, and most importantly, wearing masks need not be and should not be onerous.

In summary, until there are medications that can cure COVID-19 patients of the disease or a safe and effective vaccine is easily and widely available to provide immunity against this highly infectious disease with potentially devastating consequences, we all have to come together to beat back this virus.

Until the absence of cure, prevention is the only option, not just the best option.

To beat back the virus and not let it lock us down, get us sick or cause more deaths, we have to wear a mask, wash our hands, enjoy the outdoors, and practice physical distancing.

This will help us get back to work, get children and teachers back to school and help us get back to business and restart the US economy while we wait for a cure or a vaccine or both.

The alternative is and should not be acceptable to most, if not all. To place it in context, let us look at the alternative.

The reproduction number (R0) "estimates of the virus that causes COVID-19 ranged from 1.5 to 6.49, with a mean of 3.28 and a median of 2.79." This means that one person with COVID-19 can infect approximately 3 other people. By comparison, the R0 of the seasonal flu is 1.3 which means that one person with the seasonal flu can infect approximately 1 other person. It became known that although "asymptomatic patients with COVID-19 have a lower viral load, they still have certain period of viral shedding, which suggests the possibility of transmission during their asymptomatic period." In addition, people who are infected by the COVID-19 virus begin shedding the virus through their mouth and nose while breathing, coughing or sneezing about 2–3 days before the onset of symptoms, with the maximum shedding of the virus the day before the beginning of symptoms.

It has been thought that asymptomatic and mainly "pre-symptomatic virus shedding is thus likely a major contributor to global COVID-19 spreading as it occurs undetected under the current limited testing practice." As stated earlier, about 80% of the people who carry the virus and are asymptomatic or mildly symptomatic are responsible for almost half (44%) of all transmission even before they "become aware of carrying the disease." This makes it difficult and almost impossible to trace COVID-19 without appropriate testing.

It is obvious from the above that a coordinated and concerted plan that is applicable and followed by all of us together is what is the need of the hour if we want to beat back this pandemic.

Directly Observed Self-isolation and Contact Tracing (DOS-CT)

We can learn from our past experiences and history to do so. One of our success stories, the lessons from which can now be applied to COVID-19, is the Directly Observed Therapy (DOT) that was used so effectively to combat the Tuberculosis (TB) epidemic in New York in the 1990s as well as around the world since.

As per the CDC's own website, *"Directly observed therapy (DOT) is a key element of TB case management. Endorsed by the World Health*

COVIDSLAYERS

Organization and CDC, DOT entails a trained observer watching as the patient swallows the anti TB medications."

For those who may not be aware or recall, DOT was successfully implemented in New York for all TB patients in New York state to combat the TB epidemic in the 1990s. It is known that "drug-susceptible TB can be successfully treated with current first line anti-TB therapy…..with cure rates exceeding 95% among patients who adhere to treatment." Despite such a high success rate, Tuberculosis remains one of the leading causes of infectious disease related death worldwide with 1.3 million people dying in the year 2016. "From 1978 through 1992 the number of patients with tuberculosis in New York City nearly tripled, and the proportion of such patients who had drug resistant… tuberculosis more than doubled." Treatment of tuberculosis is long and requires taking multiple medications for a duration of at least six months. Not surprisingly, in patients who are not strictly adherent to treatment protocols, the successful cure of TB can be compromised by poor adherence. "Studies have shown the main reason TB patients relapsed, failed treatment, or become drug resistant is that they don't take their TB medications as prescribed."

In addition, patients may also develop drug resistant tuberculosis due to insufficient treatment. "The treatment for multidrug-resistant tuberculosis is difficult due to side-effects and a treatment duration of up to 3 years, which is also more expensive and often unsuccessful." Prior to the resurgence of tuberculosis in New York City, there was an increase in tuberculosis cases in the 1980s in the U.S. However, "in contrast to the national TB upswing during the 1980s, Baltimore experienced a substantial decline in TB following implementation of community – based DOT, despite highly prevalent medical social risk factors. Directly observed therapy facilitated high treatment completion rates and bacteriological evidence of cure."

A similar program was started in New York State to combat the resurgence of TB in New York. "NYC provided a prime example of a city with both increased incidence and prevalence of TB and increased rates of drug resistance." "After an increase in the number of cases of tuberculosis, New York City passed regulations to address the problem of nonadherence to treatment regiments. The commissioner of health could issue orders compelling a person to be examined for tuberculosis, to complete treatment, to receive treatment under direct observation, or to be detained for treatment." As per a study in the New England Journal of Medicine of February 4, 1999, "For most patients with tuberculosis, even those with severe social problems, completion of treatment can usually be achieved without regulatory intervention. Patients were detained on the basis of their history of tuberculosis, rather than on the basis of their social characteristics, and the less restrictive measure of mandatory directly observed therapy was often effective."

In addition to significantly decreasing the incidence and prevalence of TB in New York, the program also proved to be cost effective. In spite of initial investment which may be large based upon the number of people, DOT has been proven to be cost effective. DOT is now the standard for treatment worldwide. Investment in and "implementation of solid public health and treatment practices" helped to make the program a success.

Each patient was assigned a worker for one-to-one care. The DOT worker would go to a patient's home or work site to facilitate the process of taking medications while maintaining patient confidentiality. As a result, adherence to treatment protocol and compliance was made sure for the duration of the treatment which was about six months. This led to a high cure rate and less development of drug resistant TB.

According to the Institute of Medicine, "the most effective way of ensuring that patients are taking their medications is to use directly observed therapy, which involves having a member of the health care team observe the patient take each dose of each drug." As per a recent study, video-observed therapy (VOT) was found to be "simple" and "a viable and improved evolution of DOT." In addition, it was cost-effective and more convenient for the patient and the healthcare workers. A similar program using a computer, tablet or a cellphone with video capability called electronic DOT, or eDOT, has had successful studies.

If such an extensive program was a success in controlling the TB epidemic in New York, Baltimore and other places in the U.S., a less extensive version of it can therefore be considered for the control and mitigation of other infectious diseases, especially if there is a pandemic. In fact, the DOT program for TB is labor intensive with a requirement of persistence and resources over a period of 6 months per patient. The control and mitigation of the COVID-19 pandemic requires significantly less resources and will be significantly less labor intensive with less requirements.

A COVID-19 directly observed self-isolation and contact tracing (DOS-CT) program should last for only about 14 days per COVID-19 positive person as compared to the duration of 6 months in DOT for TB patients which is currently being practiced. Therefore, a COVID-19 containment and mitigation strategy will be less time consuming and very importantly, for a significantly less time period.

From a civil liberties perspective, wearing a mask, testing people for COVID-19, self-isolation, and contact tracing are significantly less intrusive and for a significantly shorter period of time than DOT, which is currently in practice not only in every town and state throughout the U.S. but throughout the world. DOT for TB patients is currently in practice everywhere in the U.S., and TB patients are being observed while taking their multiple pills to combat TB by a case worker – at their homes or even at their places of work. There does not obviously seem to be a call to arms or resistance to protect civil liberties and freedom against an ongoing DOT program that has been in existence since the 1990s and for the past almost 30 years.

Therefore, if DOT can not only be tolerated, but widely accepted and embraced by the American people for the mitigation of TB, then it is not inconceivable that the same American people, when appropriately and similarly educated and approached, would widely embrace a similar and less intrusive plan for the mitigation of COVID-19 which has caused so much death and destruction to their everyday lives, livelihoods, well-being and the country's economy.

It should be abundantly clear and obvious to all of us Americans by now, as well as to the administrators and policymakers, that until COVID-19 is defeated or at least significantly contained, we all will be forced by this evil into leading compromised lives, with compromised livelihoods and a compromised economy in one form or another.

In fact, taking lessons from the DOT program's success, a smart implementation of a similar program for COVID-19 – DOS-CT or eDOS-CT, in addition to saving American lives, would also facilitate in the early return of jobs, livelihoods, schools, sports, other activities, businesses and the US economy.

A patient who would get exposed and infected by the virus causing COVID-19 after being tested and identified by a positive test should be placed in isolation for 14 days. Such a patient, if remains asymptomatic should remain in home isolation for 14 days. The patient would be assigned a case worker who could then make sure that the patient does adhere to self-isolation. This would be for only 14 days. As an alternative to random daily visits by the case worker for physically confirming that the asymptomatic COVID-19 patient is adhering to isolation protocol, technology with video capability can be leveraged which is readily available for remote monitoring.

In addition, the case worker would contact trace any other individual or individuals who would have been exposed to the asymptomatic patient. All the individuals would then get tested and placed in isolation for 14 days. If the individuals test negative for the virus as per the disease progression pathophysiology of the virus, then isolation would be discontinued. With a ubiquitous presence of video capable electronic devices including hand-held devices, an electronic version of DOS-CT, or eDOS-CT, can be implemented.

If patients are symptomatic after being tested positive for COVID-19, they should then be given supportive care and treatment early and as per physician assessment in a hospital. Additional treatments and supportive care as and when they become available should be provided to all patients. The flawed direction that has been given to the public so far, to not seek medical attention until they are severely sick, should be reversed. Patients infected and diagnosed with COVID-19, even with mild symptoms, should seek early medical management rather than late.

COVIDSLAYERS

It should be the physicians who should decide which patients require treatments and when, and not administrators and politicians who appear to be more concerned about hospitals, money, their own jobs and "resources" and place them as higher priorities and above the lives and well-being of everyday Americans.

All symptomatic (including those with mild and moderate symptoms) patients should be under medical care, in isolation and managed with currently available supportive care and treatment options until they are stable and safe to be discharged with pertinent self-isolation if indicated. Antibody tests can be used in combination to assess infectivity status. It is important that patients who become asymptomatic and are stable for discharge either have a negative test result for the virus causing COVID-19 prior to discharge or are assessed for antibodies to confirm their status of infection or self-isolate themselves post-discharge for the recommended duration, so that they do not infect others. A similar model was successful in Shanghai, China.

One of the reasons why there has been a significantly high mortality among Americans is the flawed recommendation by administrators and healthcare policymakers and a resultant practice of not seeking medical attention until COVID-19 patients have significantly deteriorated. This obviously has not been the fault of everyday Americans nor due to their own personal preference or thought process.

Unfortunately, Americans so far have been misguided and advised incorrectly to seek medical attention only when they are severely sick and often when it is too late. Another reason has been inadequate testing precluding early identification of COVID-19 patients. If these patients are identified early and especially if they are symptomatic including being mildly symptomatic, then they could benefit from early management strategies which could decrease their risk of deteriorating.

A rising challenge is the random, inappropriate, and misguided use and waste of COVID-19 tests ascribed to the disingenuity, convenient opportunism and lack of medical knowledge of healthcare administrators.

Until recently, there has been a significant shortage of COVID-19 tests. Now when more tests are being made available, these COVID-19 tests, instead of being used to diagnose, isolate and contact trace, are being used indiscriminately.

More COVID-19 tests are being done on people that are not associated with any contact tracing in a random and frequent manner, with less scientific rationale and coherent strategy, and more as a revenue generating opportunity. As per news reports and word of mouth, healthcare entities appear to be indulging in profiting from COVID-19 tests by performing more outpatient tests which result in more money in the bank for these entities. As these healthcare facilities are not held responsible for the isolation or contact tracing of any patient who may have tested positive for COVID-19, they may very well be doing an indiscriminate number of COVID-19 tests while continuing to get paid for each one of those tests with no questions asked.

We have gone from an extreme of limited test availability to indiscriminate and incoherent testing. Sadly, all this while the virus keeps spreading and people continue to get infected.

It is time to let the American people know the truth! Let us all return to reality and summon courage to face the truth head-on. Americans can handle the truth! Truth makes us better and stronger – which is what is going to help us vanquish COVID-19.

COVIDSLAYERS

Dr. Rajesh Mohan

Chapter Eleven

Let us Fix It – It is about time!

There is no reason that more than 9 months after the initial assault by the pandemic, we still have not been able to control and mitigate this virus that causes COVID-19.

There is no reason that after 9 months, nurses and physicians and other frontline healthcare personnel still do not have easy provision of on demand availability of N95 masks and appropriate PPE.

There is no reason that after 9 months, nurses, doctors and other healthcare personnel still have to reprocess their N95 masks and use them multiple times.

There is no reason that even after more than 9 months, hospitals do not have readily available rapid diagnostic COVID-19 tests. There is no reason that while NBA, NFL, college football teams and other professional sports teams have unlimited and freely available COVID-19 tests for testing their athletes and support personnel every day, tests are rationed for patients in the ER of hospitals. While anyone in professional sports can get a test when they want one, the same is limited to symptomatic or suspected COVID-19 patients in many ERs.

There is no reason that more than 9 months later, in addition to COVID-19 test being limited, most test results are obtained in 24 hours or more.

COVIDSLAYERS

There is no reason that more than 9 months later, many hospitals are still not able to procure capabilities to perform rapid in house COVID-19 test which can provide results within a couple of hours at most.

There is no reason that more than 9 months later, rapid saliva tests for COVID-19 are not available in hospitals and other healthcare entities but are available for professional sports personnel and university students.

There is no reason that more than 9 months later, COVID-19 antibody tests (IgG and IgM) are not routinely available to assess the immune response of a patient infected by the virus.

There is no reason that more than 9 months later, medications and therapeutics are still rationed, and physicians are being restricted in many instances the freedom to use the full gamut of arsenal that should be readily available in their armamentarium for the benefit of their patients.

All this is despite the fact that the technology is available, and resources can be acquired.

We now know why we are in a worse situation than we should have been. We also know that we have done a worse job than many developed countries. We also know that a combination of arrogance and ignorance at multiple levels of the government–state and national, and in the bureaucracies of hospitals and healthcare institutions have impeded the ability and efforts of physicians and nurses to combat the virus and the pandemic more effectively. We are now acutely aware, more than ever, that there are inefficiencies and incompetence which are systemic in the administration of the U.S. healthcare system. The myriad of problems which have been so blatantly exposed by the pandemic are a testament to an unhealthy U.S. healthcare system.

We also know that the manner in which physicians, nurses and the frontline healthcare personnel have responded to this once-in-a-100-year pandemic, that we have hope, and that we can fix the system and make it stronger and better.

The disingenuity of the public officials, health officials, administrators and failed policymakers in leadership positions is brazenly exhibited by them in the so-called "hot washes" conducted after the initial surge of the pandemic. These are tried and tested dishonest practices of the corporate world. Quite often, these so- called "hot washes" are used by corporates to hide failures and incompetence and sweep them under the rug, absolving themselves of any accountability.

This is done by corporate administrators who take disadvantage of the goodness of people, a deep-seated ability of most people to forget and forgive, and an unwillingness by most people to dwell on tragic and difficult events with a willingness to move on.

Many times, the helplessness of employees due to the fear of losing their jobs or being branded as "difficult" employees if they do speak up restrains them and results in the administrators being let go scot-free, unscathed while being absolved of any accountability. The so-called hot wash, or "hog-wash," as I call it, is just a blatant attempt to cover up.

It is the same practice of zero accountability that we all saw after the banking crisis, which is now, in motion in healthcare.

It is well known that the field hospitals that were opened were an abject failure. It was reported that a $52 million field hospital in New York treated only 79 COVID-19 patients. Similar failures of field hospitals were seen in other states costing millions of dollars. All those millions of dollars could have been used to hire people and ramp up manufacturing of N95 masks, other PPE, and COVID-19 tests, especially with unemployment in the double digits at the time, and millions of Americans being jobless. I wonder what the "hog-wash" of these looked like!

It is a disgrace that after the initial surge of the pandemic in the US with hundreds of thousands of preventable loss of American lives with the pandemic currently showing no signs of being contained, there is a hastiness and impatience among healthcare administrators and the political leadership to "move on" and get back to "normal business."

This impatience and hastiness are essentially driven by money rather than an interest in patient care. Healthcare administrators are clamoring to get back to increasing their outpatient business so as to be able to get back to making profits. This includes outpatient surgeries or same day surgeries, outpatient testing services and discharging patients earlier than it may be optimal with a concomitant push to schedule outpatient tests for the same patients which they may have had while they were in the hospital. The way the healthcare and hospital industry has unfortunately evolved and is now mostly structured is that most hospitals, if not all, make most of their money from outpatient business rather than in-house patient care.

In the middle of a deadly pandemic, instead of using rapid COVID-19 tests to drive revenue generation, these tests should first be used by hospitals and healthcare entities by setting up testing centers in coordination with local communities, identifying asymptomatic and mildly symptomatic patients, and providing early management to symptomatic patients with recommendations of self-isolation and contact tracing to all who test positive. With a patient-centered plan, taking care of patients earlier rather than later, we will probably have less spread of the virus and fewer people will be hospitalized and die. We would, as a result, be in a much better place.

It is unfortunate that hospitals, which were initially built to take care of patients who could not be taken care of at home or as outpatients, are now looking to expand their outpatient business and decrease in-house patient care responsibilities and services. This is occurring even when most people in the U.S. are fearfully anticipating a second wave or a second surge of the pandemic going into the fall and winter.

Therefore, so that we do not commit the same mistakes again and are not placed again in a situation that is handicapped by the incompetence and disingenuity of administrators and public officials, I believe that this challenging time during this pandemic which has exposed a broken system is the ideal time to make systemic changes to healthcare administration. This challenge has provided us the opportunity to make our healthcare system better so as to be able to better serve the American people.

Taking bold, courageous, smart, and audacious actions will serve two purposes simultaneously – vanquish the COVID-19 pandemic and fix our healthcare system.

We Americans are bold, courageous, smart, and audacious. We can do this. We must do this.

Dr. Rajesh Mohan

This would not only help in the immediate containment and mitigation of the pandemic but also prevent the pandemic to continue to create havoc not only in personal but our economic lives as well.

The Influenza pandemic of 1918 had a terrible and tragic second wave which was deadlier than the first wave.

In addition, many people forget or are unaware that there was also a third wave of the 1918 Influenza pandemic which was deadlier than the first wave.

The first wave of the pandemic was in the spring of 1918 and started in March 1918. The second wave was in the fall of 1918, when it reached its peak in the US. The third wave continued into the winter of 1918 and spring of 1919 which had a worse peak than the first wave.

The second and the third wave caused more deaths than the first wave.

The pandemic eventually subsided in the summer of 1919. In addition, the1918 Influenza pandemic lasted for about 2 years throughout the world.

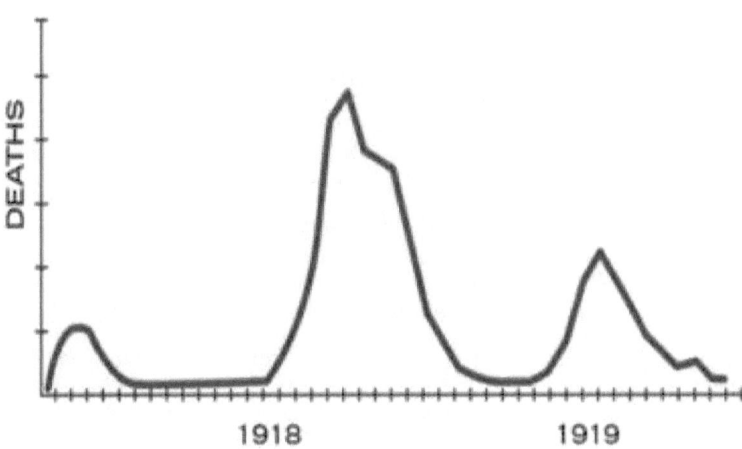

www.cdc.gov/flu/pandemic-resources/1918-commemoration/images/death-chart.jpg.

COVIDSLAYERS

It is not necessary that the COVID-19 pandemic would follow the same pattern as the 1918 Influenza pandemic.

It could be better, or it could be worse.

Although the heroic work of the doctors and nurses continues, we cannot depend on drug cures or vaccines to eradicate COVID-19 or make it inconsequential in the next six months or even a year. If miracles do happen, it would be great. If they do not, then in addition to the over 240,000 American lives lost in about 9 months, many more precious American lives tragically will continue to be added to that number.

In addition to the lives that may be tragically lost if the pandemic is not controlled, restrictions to our daily lives and livelihoods would continue in some form or the other. Some days and weeks may be better, and some days and weeks could be worse.

Most if not all of this – loss of lives and loss of livelihoods – can be prevented.

So the choice is clear – if we want less preventable American lives lost and if we want to go back to having livelihoods and open our economy anywhere near what it used to be before the pandemic, then it is essential that we control and defeat the pandemic – quickly.

For this to occur, people with demonstrable competence who know what they are doing, including having had the experience on the frontlines managing COVID-19 patients and this pandemic, and who have patients and healthcare personnel as their top priority, should be making decisions as well as making policies to combat this pandemic.

The sophistication and efficiency required to do the right thing for patients lacks among well-intentioned non-clinicians due to inadequate education and learning of medicine, experience in clinical care, as well as emotional intelligence that is so essential to create good healthcare policies and patient-centric clinical delivery models.

No matter how well-intentioned the non-clinical administrators and policymakers may be, with their primary focus and priority being *corporate health*, the required outlook towards healthcare that they possess is mostly transactional (with limited or no medical knowledge, training and experience in patient care) compared to what is actually required to efficiently provide and deliver healthcare. These mostly well-intentioned individuals are then hitched to the power of the purse string as well as administrative power – which is hard to let go even when they are out of their depths.

As per Gary S. Kaplan, MD, the chairman and CEO of Virginia Mason health system in Seattle, "When leading change, understanding the challenges and opportunities for clinical care teams at a deep level allows us to emphasize the priorities of quality, safety and respect for patients as well as care teams." He goes on to say that "in today's environment, having a physician at the most senior levels of leadership certainly helps change management and organizational success."

Physicians, nurses and clinicians who are actively involved in patient care (not retired or those who want to quit clinical practice and are looking for second careers) are the ones who should really have the power of the purse string as well as administrative power.

Physicians and clinicians who have worked for years in the healthcare profession which requires unique education, training and capabilities have developed unique abilities as a result, which no one else can possibly imbibe in a short period of time, especially during a pandemic or a crisis situation. In addition, physicians, and clinicians, through their education, training, and experience, acquire a deep knowledge about the business of their profession and their organizations including hospitals as well as the communities that they serve. The trust, the respect, and the close relationships that are built over time provide stakeholders a level of confidence in these clinical leaders which is difficult to match. This in turn has a potential to result in more beneficial strategic initiatives and decision making.

There is a myth that physicians do not understand the business of medicine and are financially irresponsible and therefore should not be in leadership management positions in healthcare.

COVIDSLAYERS

The fact is that physicians have been operating private practices and other medical entities of varying sizes and have managed them extremely well as small and medium-size businesses. Most private medical practices *are* small and medium-size businesses. And there are hundreds and thousands of them! Most of these medical practices have operated successfully, both professionally and financially, despite multiple and ever-increasing regulations and changing healthcare dynamics.

Another myth that has been propagated as a reason to keep physicians and clinical leaders away from healthcare administration and policy making is – conflict of interest.

This myth is so jarring that most people are blinded to the obvious. Administrators who are not active clinical healthcare personnel are in healthcare mainly for a job and bluntly speaking to have a livelihood and make money. Physicians, nurses, and clinical healthcare personnel who take direct clinical care of patients that are sick and come to the hospital seeking help, seek their profession mainly and mostly propelled by their conscience and passion to serve. Patient care is their primary focus and priority, providing the sick and dying, joy and more precious moments in this life on planet Earth. They do get reimbursed for their hard work which, for the most part, cannot ever have a value that is adequate or appropriate enough.

Any healthcare system and its policy's first and foremost mission has to be to provide quality patient care. It should not and must not be to line the pockets of hospitals, administrators, and the insurance industry in the garb of maintaining "financial viability" of these entities and groups of individuals.

The quality of patient care should be determined by physicians and clinical leaders and not by non-physician administrators and policymakers who tie quality of patient care to financial incentives rather than tying quality of patient care to the level and ease of patient services available to patients coming through the doors of a healthcare entity, whether it is a hospital or an outpatient center.

It is the ease and availability of patient services to patients in a timely manner that directly leads to better patient outcomes. For example, if a patient is rushed to an ER after getting his finger cut in an accident and there is no hand surgeon on staff in that hospital, then the patient would have to be transferred to another hospital which has a hand surgeon that may cause an unfavorable outcome due to the associated delay in timely surgery that may be needed, resulting in poor quality of patient care as a result. Similarly, if a patient is brought to an ER with chest pain and is found to have a heart attack and there is no cardiac catheterization available in that hospital, then the patient would have to be transferred to another hospital which has cardiac catheterization available. The associated delay in care due to the lack of timely treatment could potentially lead to less than optimal outcome, resulting in poor quality of patient care as a result.

Patient care services at most hospitals are made available determined mainly by the potential for profitability for a hospital by a patient care service as determined by administrators rather than a goal to provide patient care and the best possible patient care service for the community that a hospital is supposed to serve. Hospital financial administrators have determined that they can make more money and become more profitable if they invest more in outpatient services and cut back on in-patient services.

Currently the ease and availability of patient services in a timely manner, especially in-patient services to patients, are the biggest challenges facing patients when they seek care that may require admission to a hospital.

Since many hospitals over the years have scaled back and curtailed patient care services, especially in-patient services, it has made it harder for physicians and nurses to take care of patients as they should and would, resulting in patient outcomes that could have been better.

The poor strategic planning by mostly non-clinical financial administrators of the U.S. healthcare system have resulted in many hospitals providing inadequate and less patient-care services, primarily driven by profitability and not patient-centric care or the conviction of serving their communities.

Most among the general public including the members of local communities that many such hospitals are located in and are supposed to serve are largely unaware of the profit driven foundation on which major healthcare decisions are made. This current state of a compromised U.S. healthcare system resulting in compromised availability of patient services is a result of cost-cutting measures, incompetent management, strategy, and planning by non-clinical administrators who approach healthcare primarily from a financial and economical perspective.

I have firmly believed that in healthcare, if patients are our central focus – which they should be – and all our efforts are directed towards providing the best possible patient care in an efficient and timely manner, then the finances and the economics of healthcare would be proficient as well.

If a hospital cannot provide patient care services when needed for the community, which it is supposed to serve, resulting in the people form those communities to seek medical care in other hospitals located in other communities, then there is no reason for that hospital to exist and waste tax payer money and give a false sense of security to the members of that community.

Of course, clinical leaders do not expect hospitals to be run into the ground by a gross mismanagement of funds, or by following a haphazard and impractical approach to healthcare. Indeed, a well-run hospital needs to be profitable, thereby allowing it to provide its patients the most innovative medical treatment by a team of well-qualified medical professionals. However, myopic profitability should not be the main driving force steering hospital and healthcare administration and all their decisions.

In fact, COVID-19 has exposed the mismanagement, lack of financial alacrity and agility, and hypocrisy of many healthcare administrators resulting in limited capabilities of providing appropriate patient care. As a result, many hospitals throughout the country have started closing down.

During the current COVID-19 pandemic, our unhealthy healthcare system has resulted in and laid bare the following –

1. Lack of readily available COVID-19 diagnostic tests.
2. Lack of readily available COVID-19 antibody tests.

3. Lack of N95 masks, PAPR and other PPE.
4. Lack of securing adequate critical care nurse staffing when needed.
5. Lack of securing adequate intensivists and physicians when needed.
6. Lack of securing respiratory therapists when needed.
7. Lack of securing adequate nurses aids when needed.
8. Lack of procuring adequate medications when needed.
9. Lack of adequate local stockpile of essential resources and materials.
10. Lack of realistic financial planning for immediate, short-term, and long-term contingencies.
11. Lack of access to appropriate patient care services for patients requiring hospital care with medical conditions other than COVID-19.
12. Lack of ability to improvise and adapt, resulting in the curtailment or stoppage of patient care services.
13. Lack of flexibility to adapt due to ingrained dogmas perpetuating conformity for corporate benefit rather than patient benefit.
14. Lack of ability to work with communities that are supposed to be served due to barriers in place that intentionally or unintentionally impede efforts.
15. Lack of presence of actively practicing physicians at the top levels of hospital and healthcare leadership – some hospitals and healthcare systems did better (e.g. – Mount Sinai, NY, Mayo Clinic, MN).
16. Lack of capabilities with a possible associated insecurity among healthcare administrators, resulting in the minimal involvement and presence of not only qualified but competent actively

practicing physicians and clinical leaders in policy and decision making, relating to the pandemic.

17. Lack of leadership and knowledge among most healthcare administrators resulting in not recognizing (or not wanting to recognize) the crisis early or adequately enough, resulting in inadequate outreach, education, and collaboration with political leaders. This resulted in a poor public health policy locally in communities, county, state, and national level, if any.
18. Lack of a cohesive testing, isolation, contact tracing and hospital admission strategy and planning at every local community level.
19. Lack of consistency in recommendations and guidelines based upon science and full transparency rather than convenience.
20. Lack of trust in healthcare administrative leaders.

When corporate welfare takes precedence over patient welfare, such a healthcare system is doomed for failure.

When profiting is more important than patient life and well-being, such a healthcare system is doomed for failure. When crunching numbers for the benefit of the insurance industry, hospitals and drug industry is more important than finding ways to increase the capability to provide health care to sick people, the healthcare system is doomed for failure.

Therefore, most of the non-clinical administrators, public officials and policymakers in healthcare should collaborate with actively *practicing* physicians and clinical leaders. These clinical leaders should then be empowered to make decisions regarding resources, strategies and the development and implementation of policies as they may deem appropriate during this war against a once-in-a-100-years pandemic.

Once this war is won, then the lessons learned should be implemented in the development of a "new" healthcare system which is robust, flexible, and dynamic – all at the same time.

Dr. Rajesh Mohan

A "new" healthcare system would place patient care first and not corporate care and fealty.

A successful "new" healthcare system will be one when it achieves the trust of the people and the communities that it serves.

A successful "new" healthcare system will be one when the leaders who lead the healthcare system gain the trust of not only the people and communities that they serve but the employees, the physicians, the nurses and all healthcare personnel who make the healthcare system.

What needs to be done initially as a minimum in order to give an impetus to reinvigorate and reset our war against the COVID-19 pandemic are the following –

1. Ramping up the availability of same day COVID-19 diagnostic tests.
2. Ramping up the availability of same day COVID-19 antibody test.
3. Easy and barrier free availability of N95 masks and other PPE outside patient rooms.
4. Make sure there is adequate nurse staffing, especially critical care, with a robust bench strength based upon frequent, periodic assessment so as to avoid panic, unavailability, or compromise in patient care in crisis or surge situations.
5. Make sure there is adequate intensivist and physician staffing, with a robust bench strength based upon frequent, periodic assessment so as to avoid panic, unavailability, or compromise in patient care in crisis or surge situations.
6. Make sure there are adequate respiratory therapists, with a robust bench strength based upon frequent, periodic assessment so as to avoid panic, unavailability, or compromise in patient care in crisis or surge situations.
7. Make sure there are adequate nurses aids, with a robust bench strength based upon frequent, periodic assessment so as to avoid

panic, unavailability, or compromise in patient care in crisis or surge situations.

8. Make sure there is an adequate stock of in-house medications with a sufficient local back up stockpile based upon frequent, periodic assessment so as to avoid panic, unavailability, or compromise in patient care in crisis or surge situations.

9. Make sure there is adequate local stockpile of essential resources and materials based upon frequent, periodic assessment so as to avoid panic, unavailability, or compromise in patient care in crisis or surge situations.

10. Make sure there is a cohesive testing, isolation, contact tracing and hospital admission strategy and plan at every local community led by science and developed by a collaboration between local political and administrative leaders and the clinical physician administrative leaders representing hospitals and healthcare systems.

11. Collaboration between all statewide and nationwide clinical physician administrative leaders to develop consistent recommendations and guidelines based upon science with full transparency.

12. Make sure there is robust financial planning with frequent, periodic assessment so as to avoid panic, unavailability, or compromise in patient care in crisis or surge situations.

13. Make sure there are patient services available, even during crisis or surge situations, with a frequent, periodic assessment so as to avoid panic, unavailability, or compromise in patient care in crisis or surge situations.

14. Make sure there is flexibility to adapt to unexpected situations with the goal being to avoid disruption in the continuation of patient care services in a safe way.

15. Recruitment and placement of practicing physicians in leadership and administrative positions in hospitals and across the healthcare system.

16. Science based development and implementation of policies and healthcare administrative decisions by physicians who are in administrative leadership positions and continue to provide clinical patient care.

17. Collaboration with political leaders at local, state, and national levels, to educate and develop public health policies based upon science and led by clinical physician administrative leaders serving as representatives of hospitals and healthcare systems.

18. Collaboration between political leadership at community, state and national level and clinical physician administrative leaders of hospital and healthcare systems to develop guidance based upon science to efficiently and safely restart and rejuvenate businesses and open schools so as to encourage and revitalize economic growth.

19. Collaboration between political leadership and clinical physician administrative leaders of hospitals and healthcare systems to facilitate development of safe medications, therapeutics, and vaccines by scientists so as to make them readily available to all Americans in a safe and transparent manner without jeopardizing their safety.

20. If all of the above is done in a systematic and sustained manner with systemic changes occurring for the most part organically and simultaneously, then there will be a development of trust in our healthcare leaders and in our healthcare system. The trust and goodwill generated as a result will increase and improve compliance to health-related recommendations by such healthcare entities and healthcare leaders leading to improved health and well-being of our people and communities.

If we genuinely care about our fellow Americans and fellow humans, we have to stop waiting for things to get better on their own or that someone else will do it for us, hoping that COVID-19 (in the future it may be something else) does not come close to home – of any and all Americans. We have no better choice than to begin on the righteous path, traveled only by the brave and the courageous, in earnest. We have no choice other than a comprehensive and a rapid dominance strategy to vanquish this pandemic. This is similar to the shock and awe doctrine that is applied by the U.S. military.

We are at war against COVID-19 in this pandemic. Americans do not get defeated, by anyone or anything. We have to win this war. There is no other option.

So why go piecemeal and small?

Let us go BIG!!

Dr. Rajesh Mohan

Chapter Twelve

The Warriors, The Martyrs - All Heroes

There are innumerable, and untold stories of valor, strength, fortitude, and sacrifice that have in many cases become folklore at battlegrounds called hospitals in local communities across the U.S. and the world.

COVID-19, as a mortal risk for healthcare providers themselves, and their families, was not one that anyone was prepared for. Physicians and nurses and other healthcare personnel have always risen to the challenge of curing patients with the deadliest of diseases in the past. The risk of personally getting infected and succumbing to an infectious agent has never been this high and with this ease.

The joy of waking up in the morning and embarking on a mission to make people better has never been tempered so much by the risk of mortality, one's own mortality. The joy of the ride back home after a successful day or night after making a positive difference in people's lives has never been tempered so much by the fear of possibly transmitting the deadly virus to one's own family members.

It is one thing to place one's own life and health at risk in the battle against a highly infectious disease in the service of patients. It is another to place your family members' lives and health at risk as well – a terrifying proposition that every healthcare personnel struggled(s) with every day.

The daily routine of undressing in the garage and hurriedly walking to the bathroom like an untouchable to cleanse oneself intentionally so as to remove any speck of the invisible virus that may have found a place to thrive on the bodies of the warriors has been demeaning, disheartening and rankling – all at the same time. It has bewildered many that a virus which can easily be disintegrated and destroyed by soap and water and proper hygiene, as long as it does not gain access into a human body, would be the cause of so much havoc and so many deaths.

"Don't be a hero," said my younger brother in a phone conversation in the midst of the pandemic. "But I know you are going to do what you have to do and will not listen to me," he followed. He has known me since he was born and knows me too well. There is no way that I would be sitting at home and not join in the fight of a century, and take a back seat.

This, I am sure, has been the conversation in almost every healthcare professional's home and with their loved ones. Healthcare professionals who continue to fight on the frontlines in the service of humanity, placing themselves at risk at all times, especially during this lethal pandemic, are a special breed of humans. This pandemic presented a historic moment that no physician or nurse who took to the healthcare profession as a calling could or would refuse to engage in, despite the risk the virus posed to them. The humility and the sense of service is so pronounced in them that, accolades notwithstanding, the will to be a part of something larger than themselves drives them to overcome seemingly insurmountable heights of fear and challenge.

Nurses, physicians, and respiratory therapists have stepped into patient rooms innumerable times to provide resuscitation and intubation to crashing patients, mindful of the associated risk, along with the fear of getting infected hovering over their own existence.

Nurses have held the hands of dying patients infected with COVID-19 until they felt the power of life leave those hands. They have then wept alone and tried to overcome the sorrow only loved ones would know – because they were the loved ones of those patients, in those last moments. They made sure that no patient died alone.

Intensivists, anesthesiologists, and respiratory therapists would frequently be intubating patients and connecting them to ventilators in rooms with air that was infested with the virus, not knowing who among them would be the next victim, in a potentially deadly Russian roulette gone viral.

Environmental services personnel would try to cover themselves as much as they could and hope that in the process of getting rid of the deadly virus from every corner and crevice in a room, no amount of the invisible virus takes a ride with them back home which could result in tragedy and death.

Physicians of all kinds - ER physicians, infectious disease, cardiologists, nephrologists, internal medicine, surgeons, radiologists, pulmonologists, hematologists, and others would mostly flock towards their duty and responsibility to care for patients. Many even came out of their retirements, placing themselves at risk even when they did not have to – because that is what they thought was the right thing to do. Many overcame their fears through their will to serve and make a difference. Most importantly, even though many private practice physicians were not bound by employment contracts or the need of a paycheck and medical insurance, they still volunteered to serve in the darkest and most challenging of times healthcare has seen in the past century.

Not everyone volunteered to become a potential willing martyr. Some employees – nurses, employed physicians and others – needed a paycheck and medical insurance. Some with risk factors, including age, decided to not take risks and hunker down. It was understandable if someone was afraid – one cannot and should not blame a person who is fearful. One cannot and should not force people to go to war if they are fearful. It was also not right to force people to put their lives at risk as well as the lives of their family members.

Healthcare warriors – the brave, the fine, the exceptional men and women – who were left to fight the war had to battle every day for long hours with an increasing workload due to staffing challenges. With more intense work in treating patients infected with COVID-19, while wearing PPE that was essential but onerous, especially when worn for long hours, nurses, physicians and other healthcare personnel galvanized superhuman courage way beyond their training to achieve exceptional and unforeseen results.

Dr. Rajesh Mohan

Until about mid-August, CDC had counted a total of 625 healthcare workers who had lost their lives during this pandemic. This number was challenged as underreported by Dr. Claire Rezba, an anesthesiologist in a hospital in Richmond, Virginia. According to her, the number of lives lost while working in healthcare were at least 1,000. More than two plane loads of American healthcare personnel have died in 9 months from this pandemic. The number has continued to increase even by CDC's count. The CDC continues to be behind in identifying the dead or alive status of all COVID-19 confirmed cases among healthcare personnel.

We should get the count right of the brave and martyred healthcare warriors so that we can at least give them the respect and admiration that they deserve.

In fact, it would only be appropriate to honor fallen healthcare warriors who gave the ultimate sacrifice, by dedicating a COVID-19 pandemic memorial to them.

COVIDSLAYERS

Dr. Rajesh Mohan

Epilogue

In battling this pandemic of COVID-19, Americans in general, and healthcare personnel in particular, have had to unfortunately follow the principle of survival of the fittest.

Young people who consider themselves invincible, sometimes to their own detriment, have so far not faced tragic consequences in large numbers. The elderly and the frail have succumbed in large numbers due to this lethal virus.

Physicians, nurses, and other healthcare personnel, through their dedication, intelligence, and diligent care of the sick and the affected, have prevented, to a large extent, this tragedy from causing an even wider scale of death and destruction. More Americans would have succumbed to the virus by now if it were not for the knowledge, skills and the ingenuity of physicians that orchestrated the materialization of innovative treatments and patient management strategies while breaking through the dogmas of prescriptive policies and protocols.

Healthcare in America should not and must not function wherein patients and healthcare personnel are battling just to survive.

It should never be left to a scenario where survival of the fittest is the only and best option, especially in the face of challenges like a pandemic.

If our healthcare system, hospitals and other entities within the system are incapable of taking care of fellow Americans, especially when times are tough and the need is most, such as during a pandemic, then what is the use of such a healthcare system?

In the year 2018, the total cost for hospital care in the United States was about $1.2 trillion out of a total of about $3.6 trillion total US national health expenditure (NHE) according to publicly available information from the CMS.

Therefore, almost $1 out of every $3 spent on the entire NHE is spent for hospital care. And, about 25 percent of total spending on hospital care was on administrative costs.

In comparison, the 2018 United States National Defense Budget was $612 billion according to publicly available information from the US Department of Defense.

The 2018 cost for hospital care was almost twice the entire National Defense budget.

Why should the taxpayers support such a dysfunctional system when the sick and especially the elderly appear to be dispensable? Aren't Medicare dollars primarily supposed to take care of the elderly!

Many have said that the COVID-19 pandemic did not break the system; instead, it exposed a broken system.

Therefore, going forward, if we really want to progress and improve our healthcare system which everyone believes we should, then the first step must be to stop pining for the flawed system, let alone try to return to the past and business as usual. The pandemic laid bare the systemic flaws in our healthcare system which resulted in a lack of accessibility for patients seeking care as well as making it challenging for physicians and nurses to provide patient care.

The disruption that the pandemic has caused in our healthcare system has given us an opportunity to potentially transform the healthcare system into one where patient care is the culture – first and omnipresent, and not just a priority. We can channel the energy from this disruptive force to shake up, dislodge and remove the deeply embedded chronic issues in our healthcare system that have enabled the forces that resist change. A jump-start from the energy derived from this disruptive force could transform the U.S. healthcare system for the benefit of all Americans.

This jump-start should be for one purpose and one purpose only - patient care. People who want to be and are involved in this transformative process should leave their personal agendas at the door.

Dr. Rajesh Mohan

Many well-intentioned people such as Bill Gates who have abundant money and resources to spare, bring their own personal agendas along with their purported intentions to assist and improve healthcare, whenever they do so. Bill Gates, for example, instead of investing money in a vaccine developing German biotech company, could have easily invested in factories in the U.S. to make N95 masks and other PPE as well as reagents that are required for COVID-19 tests during this pandemic. These so-called philanthropic efforts of such multi-billionaires should be directed not by ROI but by interests of patients or IOP. These efforts of apparent or professed altruism, instead of being random and misdirected, should be guided by practicing clinical administrative leaders.

No matter how successful such philanthropists are, and how well intentioned they might be, they are unfortunately challenged by their lack of training and expertise from a clinical perspective. For a successful patient-centered healthcare system, clinical and business decision making expertise is required to create dynamic and efficient clinical delivery models for the benefit of patients. Therefore, the resources of philanthropists and those with humanitarian leanings would yield maximum results when done in collaboration with physician administrative leaders, lest it may just turn out to be a name on the walls of a hallway or a building.

A patient-first healthcare system would be led by practicing clinical administrative leaders. Other options that have been tried for more than a century have resulted in the current state of our stumbling healthcare system.

As per a report in 2014 by the American College of Physician Executives, only approximately 5 percent of hospital leaders are physicians. As per an article in Becker's Hospital Review, "Conventional knowledge suggests physicians should focus on clinical care while managers with business or administrative backgrounds command hospitals daily operations, but this notion is likely outdated, if not fundamentally flawed." In a study published in July 2011 by Amanda H Goodall, analyzing data collected on top 100 US hospitals and 300 chief executive officers of hospitals in the U.S., the paper found "a strong positive association between the ranked quality of a hospital and whether the CEO is a physician."

With patient-centered care as the mission of a transformed, new, and improved healthcare system, it should be apparent that practicing clinical leaders with additional expertise in the business aspect of the healthcare sector would be more effective than non-clinical leaders.

A patient-care centric healthcare system must be driven primarily from a clinical perspective. A patient-care centric clinical decision-making leader can adapt and be more nimble to free market demands, so as to make the healthcare system and its entities function more efficiently and successfully without any compromise to patient care.

Practicing clinical physician leaders have first-hand knowledge and experience with a better understanding and appreciation of the work done by the frontline staff. Challenges faced by frontline healthcare personnel are less likely to go unnoticed and unaddressed. Patient-care centered decision-making by physician leaders would be more focused and with more clarity.

A clinical leader respected amongst his or her peers has more trust and alignment with the medical and clinical staff for successful implementation of health care strategies. This would increase the probability of improving patient care, safety, and quality.

According to Donald Sull and colleagues in the March 2015 issue of the Harvard Business Review, execution of strategic objectives of a company due to lack of coordination amongst silos is a significant reason. In addition, they state that, "When managers come up with creative solutions to unforeseen problems or run with unexpected opportunities, they are not undermining systematic implementation; they are demonstrating execution at its best period." In their study, they found "that nine managers in 10 expect some of their organizations' major initiatives to fail for lack of resources." They found that "only 11% of the managers who we have surveyed believe that all their company's strategic priorities have the financial and human resources needed for success." According to their article, it was not the lack of adherence to plans, but the lack of agility that was a barrier to executing strategies successfully.

Dr. Rajesh Mohan

Strict adherence to prescriptive actions dumbs down the ability of critical thinking and facing unorthodox or unexpected situations. The hesitancy to face conflicts with the hope that prescriptive behavior would lead to resolution of unexpected and difficult challenges, promoted by most rigid corporate structures, is a lackadaisical and apathy laden approach.

Interestingly, the above appears to be true of the U.S. healthcare system as well, which the COVID-19 pandemic has exposed so blatantly. The current approach should not and cannot be persisted with in healthcare, wherein real lives are on the line every single moment.

Healthcare should be part of the national security apparatus at the highest level. A healthcare agency which would encompass the health and well-being of the American people in its entirety should have an independent seat at the table at the highest level.

Although we are currently in the midst of an infectious disease pandemic, this healthcare agency would encompass not just infectious diseases but all specialties and all facets regarding the health and well-being of all Americans. It should be led by a practicing clinical administrative physician leader.

This healthcare agency would have access to the highest level of national security and intelligence information. Similar to the National Security Agency (NSA), this healthcare agency would be responsible for the health security of all Americans, defending them from threats both external and internal, including all diseases and pandemics. It would be responsible for the coordination among various silos in the American healthcare system like the CDC, the National Institutes of health (NIH) and various other healthcare agencies.

This agency will lead the response and coordinate with all state healthcare agencies in national emergency situations when the health and well-being of the American people is on the line.

It would provide national guidelines, containment, and mitigation strategies to defeat the threats to the health and well-being of Americans.

COVIDSLAYERS

It would coordinate with scientists, physicians, the private sector, including the pharmaceutical industry, laboratory services, device manufacturers and supply chain partners.

It would ensure that the frontline healthcare personnel – boots on the ground, have all the resources to successfully combat any threats to the health and well-being of the American people.

If we really care for our own health and well-being and that of our fellow Americans, then we should go all out to vanquish COVID-19.

If we really care for our own livelihoods and the economic well-being of our fellow Americans, then we should not hold anything back to vanquish COVID-19.

If we really want to vanquish COVID-19, then we should make sure that all our frontline healthcare warriors have body armor (PPE), rapid COVID-19 tests, and all the weapons they need to be victorious.

If we really care for the economic well-being of our country and want to remain the richest, strongest and the greatest country on Earth, then we should join hands with our physicians, nurses and frontline healthcare personnel, who are leading by example, and vanquish COVID-19.

If we really want to vanquish COVID-19, then we should do what our frontline healthcare warriors are inspiring us to do.

Together we all will vanquish this pandemic and come out of this stronger and better and will rise as COVIDSLAYERS!

Dr. Rajesh Mohan

COVIDSLAYERS

Bibliography

Chapter One

The Sirens were Blaring

1. Vinessa Erminio | NJ Advance Media for NJ.com. Coronavirus in New Jersey: A timeline of the outbreak. nj. https://www.nj.com/coronavirus/2020/03/coronavirus-in-new-jersey-a-timeline-of-the-outbreak.html. Posted March 24, 2020; Published June 12, 2020.
2. Anthony G. Attrino | NJ Advance Media for NJ.com. N.J. coronavirus update: Fort Lee man, 32, is first to test positive for virus in state. nj. https://www.nj.com/coronavirus/2020/03/nj-coronavirus-update-fort-lee-man-32-is-first-to-test-positive-for-virus-in-state.html. Published March 5, 2020.
3. Official Site of The State of New Jersey. Office of the Governor | TRANSCRIPT: March 13th, 2020 Coronavirus Briefing Media. https://www.nj.gov/governer/news/news/562020/20200312b.shtml.

Chapter Two

The Real (Not the Fake) Panic

None.

Chapter Three

When the Cavalry Is Delayed – Do It Yourself – Do not Wait

None

Chapter Four

Guidelines for Convenience

and

CDC's Fall from Grace

4. Mandavilli A. How Long Will Coronavirus Live on Surfaces or in the Air Around You? The New York Times. https://www.nytimes.com/2020/03/17/health/coronavirus-surfaces-aerosols.html?action=click. Published March 17, 2020.

5. Volkin S. How long can the virus that causes COVID-19 live on surfaces? The Hub. https://hub.jhu.edu/2020/03/20/sars-cov-2-survive-on-surfaces/. Published March 20, 2020.

6. Doremalen Nvan, Bushmaker T, Morris DH, and others. Aerosol and Surface Stability of SARS-CoV-2 as Compared with SARS-CoV-1: NEJM. New England Journal of Medicine. https://www.nejm.org/doi/10.1056/NEJMc2004973. Published April 16, 2020.

7. HealthLeaders. Nearly One-Fifth of Providers Dealing With Higher Medical Mask Prices. HealthLeaders Media. https://www.healthleadersmedia.com/finance/nearly-one-fifth-providers-dealing-higher-medical-mask-prices. https://www.cdc.gov/infectioncontrol/pdf/guidelines/isolation-guidelines-H.pdf.

8. Face mask shortage prompts CDC to loosen coronavirus guidance. Home. https://www.pharmacist.com/article/face-mask-shortage-prompts-cdc-loosen-coronavirus-guidance. Published March 11, 2020.

9. Kopp E. Hospitals seek to kill a policy shielding nurses from COVID-19. Roll Call. https://rollcall.com/2020/03/13/hospitals-want-to-kill-a-policy-shielding-nurses-from-covid-19-because-there-arent-enough-masks/. Published March 13, 2020.

10. Trafton A, Chu J, Chandler DL. Covid-19 diagnostic based on MIT technology might be tested on patient samples soon. MIT News | Massachusetts Institute of Technology. https://news.mit.edu/2020/covid-19-diagnostic-test-prevention-0312. Published March 12, 2020.

11. Ariana Eunjung Cha MM. Hospital workers battling coronavirus turn to bandannas, sports goggles and homemade face shields amidshortages.TheWashingtonPost. https://www.washingtonpost.com/health/2020/03/19/hospital-workers-battling-coronavirus-turn-bandanas-sports-goggles-homemade-face-shields-amid-shortages/. Published March 19, 2020.

12. SignthePetition.Change.org. https://www.change.org/p/hospital-administrators-us-physicians-healthcare-workers-for-personal-protective-equipment-in-covid-19-pandemic.

13. Kopp E. CDC suggests nurses use bandanas, scarves during face mask shortage. https://www.rollcall.com/2020/03/18/cdc-suggests-nurses-use-bandanas-scarves-during-face-mask-shortage/. Published March 18, 2020.

14. https://www.fda.gov/files/n95_respirator.jpg. Published August 20, 2020.

15. https://www.fda.gov/files/surgical_mask_0.jpg.Published August 20, 2020.

16. https://www.cdc.gov/coronavirus/2019-ncov/images/hcp/N95-infographic-What-Are-APR-508.png?noicon.

17. Roberts V. To PAPR or not to PAPR? Canadian journal of respiratory therapy: CJRT = Revue canadienne de la therapie respiratoire:RCTR.
https://www.ncbi.nlm.nih.gov/pmc/articles/PMC4456839/. Published 2014.

18. Considerations for Optimizing the Supply of Powered Air-Purifying Respirators (PAPRs). Centers for Disease Control and Prevention.https://www.cdc.gov/coronavirus/2019-ncov/hcp/ppe-strategy/powered-air-purifying-respirators-strategy.html.

19. MarketsandMarkets. Patient Safety and Risk Management Solutions Market Worth $2.2 Billion by 2024. PR Newswire: news distribution, targeting and monitoring. https://www.prnewswire.com/news-releases/patient-safety-and-risk-management-solutions-market-worth-2-2-billion-by-2024--300906790.html. Published August 26, 2019.

Chapter Five

Science and Logic became Dispensable

20. Klar R. Hospital CEO: $7 being charged for 58-cent masks. TheHill. https://thehill.com/policy/healthcare/488408-hospital-ceo-7-being-charged-for-58-cent-masks. Published March 19, 2020.

21. Rosalsky G. Are High Mask Prices The Problem Or The Solution?NPR.
https://www.npr.org/sections/money/2020/03/03/811181309/ar

e-high-mask-prices-the-problem-or-the-solution. Published March 3, 2020.

22. Feldman A. 3M Ships More Than Half-Million N95 Masks To New York And Seattle As It Cranks Up Production. Forbes. https://www.forbes.com/sites/amyfeldman/2020/03/22/3m-ships-more-than-half-million-n95-masks-to-new-york-and-seattle-as-it-cranks-up-production/. Published March 23, 2020.

23. Nick. Top 10 N95 Mask Manufacturers in the World 2020: Coronavirus Boosts N95 Respirators Market Sales. Technavio. https://blog.technavio.com/blog/top-10-n95-mask-manufacturers. Published April 14, 2020.

24. Strategies for Optimizing the Supply of Facemasks: COVID-19. Centers for Disease Control and Prevention. https://www.cdc.gov/coronavirus/2019-ncov/hcp/ppe-strategy/face-masks.html.

25. Recommended Guidance for Extended Use and Limited Reuse of N95 Filtering Facepiece Respirators in Healthcare Settings. Centers for Disease Control and Prevention. https://www.cdc.gov/niosh/topics/hcwcontrols/recommendedguidanceextuse.html. Published March 27, 2020.

26. COVID-19 Decontamination and Reuse of Filtering Facepiece Respirators. Centers for Disease Control and Prevention. https://www.cdc.gov/coronavirus/2019-ncov/hcp/ppe-strategy/decontamination-reuse-respirators.html.

27. AirbornePrecautions.cdc.gov. https://www.cdc.gov/infectioncontrol/pdf/airborne-precautions-sign-P.pdf.

28. ContactPrecautions.cdc.gov. https://www.cdc.gov/infectioncontrol/pdf/contact-precautions-sign-P.pdf.

29. DropletPrecautions.cdc.gov. https://www.cdc.gov/infectioncontrol/pdf/droplet-precautions-sign-P.pdf.

30. Rodrigo Torrejon | NJ Advance Media for NJ.com. N.J.'s 1st major coronavirus testing site hits capacity after just 4 hours. nj. https://www.nj.com/coronavirus/2020/03/njs-1st-major-coronavirus-testing-site-hits-capacity-shuts-down-after-just-4-hours.html. Published March 20, 2020.

31. Rodrigo Torrejon | NJ Advance Media for NJ.com. Coronavirus testing site at Bergen hits capacity before opening - again. nj. https://www.nj.com/coronavirus/2020/03/coronavirus-testing-site-at-bergen-hits-capacity-before-opening-again.html. Published March 24, 2020.

32. Matthew Stanmyre | NJ Advance Media for NJ.com, NJ.com RE| F. Coronavirus testing in N.J. has been a mess from the start. Here'swhatwentwrong.nj. https://www.nj.com/coronavirus/2020/03/coronavirus-testing-in-nj-has-been-a-mess-from-the-start-heres-what-went-wrong.html. Published March 30, 2020.

Chapter Six

Misplaced Priorities – Healthcare is About Patients First, Stupid!

33. Zhou R, Li F, Chen F, et al. Viral dynamics in asymptomatic patients with COVID-19. International journal of infectious diseases : IJID : official publication of the International Society forInfectiousDiseases. https://www.ncbi.nlm.nih.gov/pmc/articles/PMC7211726/. Published July 2020.

34. Tromberg BJ, Al. E, Author AffiliationsFrom the National Institute of Biomedical Imaging and Bioengineering (B.J.T.),

Editors T, J. H. Beigel and Others, Group TRECOVERYC. Rapid Scaling Up of Covid-19 Diagnostic Testing in the United States - The NIH RADx Initiative: NEJM. New England Journal of Medicine. https://www.nejm.org/doi/full/10.1056/NEJMsr2022263. Published October 8, 2020.

35. Rodrigo Torrejon | NJ Advance Media for NJ.com. N.J.'s 1st major coronavirus testing site hits capacity after just 4 hours. nj.

36. https://www.nj.com/coronavirus/2020/03/njs-1st-major-coronavirus-testing-site-hits-capacity-shuts-down-after-just-4-hours.html. Published March 20, 2020.

37. Rodrigo Torrejon | NJ Advance Media for NJ.com. Coronavirus testing site at Bergen hits capacity before opening - again. nj. https://www.nj.com/coronavirus/2020/03/coronavirus-testing-site-at-bergen-hits-capacity-before-opening-again.html. Published March 24, 2020.

38. Matthew Stanmyre | NJ Advance Media for NJ.com, NJ.com RE| F. Coronavirus testing in N.J. has been a mess from the start. Here'swhatwentwrong.nj. https://www.nj.com/coronavirus/2020/03/coronavirus-testing-in-nj-has-been-a-mess-from-the-start-heres-what-went-wrong.html. Published March 30, 2020.

39. Nida F. Degesys MD. Correlation Between N95 Extended Use and Reuse and Fit Failure in an Emergency Department. JAMA. https://jamanetwork.com/journals/jama/fullarticle/2767023. Published July 7, 2020.

40. Degesys NF, Wang RC, Kwan E, Fahimi J, Noble JA, Raven MC. Correlation Between N95 Extended Use and Reuse and Fit FailureinanEmergencyDepartment.JAMA. https://www.ncbi.nlm.nih.gov/pmc/articles/PMC7273312/. Published July 7, 2020.

41. COVID-19 Decontamination and Reuse of Filtering Facepiece Respirators. Centers for Disease Control and Prevention.

https://www.cdc.gov/coronavirus/2019-ncov/hcp/ppe-strategy/decontamination-reuse-respirators.html.

42. Azad A, Nedelman M. Used facemasks and bandanas: How the CDC is warning hospitals to prepare for coronavirus shortages. CNN.https://www.cnn.com/2020/03/19/health/hospital-coronavirus-shortages-preparedness/index.html. Published March 19, 2020.

43. PPE composition: Variations matter. Physicians Practice. https://www.physicianspractice.com/view/ppe-composition-variations-matter?seriesVid=2

Chapter Seven

Bigotry and Humanity – In a Pandemic

44. Greenblatt JA. Blaming Jews for the spread of the coronavirus is anti-Semitism pure and simple. nydailynews.com. https://www.nydailynews.com/opinion/ny-oped-jews-coronavirus-antisemitism-20200408-4arvpei6wvd4td7eyqxpjfhaka-story.html. Published April 8, 2020.

45. Matt Arco | NJ Advance Media for NJ.com M, Amanda Hoover | NJ Advance Media For NJ.com A. 'Don't be the knucklehead who ruins it,' Murphy says. N.J. could stop reopening if coronaviruscasesspike.nj. https://www.nj.com/coronavirus/2020/06/dont-be-the-knucklehead-who-ruins-it-murphy-says-nj-could-stop-reopening-if-coronavirus-cases-spike.html. Published June 23, 2020.

46. McDonnell T. If you've recovered from Covid-19, here's one way you might be able to help others. Quartz. https://qz.com/1828563/how-to-help-others-if-youve-recovered-from-covid-19/. Published March 30, 2020.

47. Weise E, Johnson M. The first US coronavirus patients are being treated with convalescent plasma therapy. Will it work? Not eventhedoctorsknow.USAToday. https://www.usatoday.com/story/news/health/2020/04/01/coronavirus-plasma-therapy-5-us-patients-covid-19-donors/5090946002/. Published April 2, 2020.

48. Zhang S. America Needs Plasma From COVID-19 Survivors Now.TheAtlantic. https://www.theatlantic.com/science/archive/2020/03/plasma-blood-covid-19-survivors/609007/. Published May 4, 2020.

49. True claim: New York City hospital asks recovered COVID-19 patients for blood donations to help the sick. Reuters. https://www.reuters.com/article/uk-factcheck-coronavirus-mount-sinai/true-claim-new-york-city-hospital-asks-recovered-covid-19-patients-for-blood-donations-to-help-the-sick-idUSKBN21L35H. Published April 3, 2020.

50. Conor Ferguson and Cynthia McFadden and Jaime Longoria and Rich Schapiro. A COVID-19 'mitzvah': Orthodox Jews donate blood plasma by the thousands. Yahoo! News. https://news.yahoo.com/covid-19-mitzvah-orthodox-jews-124134860.html?guccounter=1. Published July 13, 2020.

51. Hoffman R. In the Blood: The Evolving Medical and Jewish Tale of COVID Plasma Treatments: Jewish Culture. Hamodia. https://hamodia.com/prime/blood-evolving-medical-jewish-tale-covid-plasma-treatments/.

52. Ackerman T. Houston Methodist first in the nation to try coronavirus blood transfusion therapy. HoustonChronicle.com. https://www.houstonchronicle.com/news/houston-texas/article/Houston-Methodist-first-in-the-nation-to-try-15164229.php. Published March 29, 2020.

53. Reynolds E. It's the worst disaster of the pandemic. But WHO chief says our lack of concern shows 'moral bankruptcy'. CNN. https://www.cnn.com/2020/09/04/health/elderly-care-

coronavirus-who-tedros-intl/index.html. Published September 4, 2020.

54. https://policyexchange.org.uk/wp-content/uploads/Australia-and-the-Coronavirus-Crisis.pdf.

Chapter Eight
The Dogma of Bureaucracy

55. Wood J. These are the world's most respected professions. World EconomicForum. https://www.weforum.org/agenda/2019/01/these-are-the-world-s-most-respected-professions/. Published January 15, 2019.

56. Borders M. The Chart that Could Undo the Healthcare System: Max Borders. FEE Freeman Article. https://fee.org/articles/the-chart-that-could-undo-the-us-healthcare-system/. Published April 29, 2015.

57. Kocher R. The Downside of Health Care Job Growth. Harvard Business Review. https://hbr.org/2013/09/the-downside-of-health-care-job-growth. Published September 23, 2013.

Chapter Nine
The Inhumane Visitors Policy

58. Dunn A. Fact check: Are coronavirus patients dying alone in hospitals?USAToday. https://www.usatoday.com/story/news/factcheck/2020/04/09/fact-check-coronavirus-patients-dying-alone-hospitals/5114282002/. Published May 1, 2020.

59. Wakam GK, Author AffiliationsFrom the Department of Surgery, Editors T, J. H. Beigel and Others, Group TRECOVERYC. Not Dying Alone - Modern Compassionate Care in the Covid-19 Pandemic: NEJM. New England Journal of Medicine. https://www.nejm.org/doi/full/10.1056/NEJMp2007781?query=featured_home. Published October 8, 2020.

60. 'Patients dying alone': The frightening reality of many COVID-19 patients' final moments. Advisory Board Daily Briefing. https://www.advisory.com/daily-briefing/2020/03/26/dying-alone.

61. Lamas DJ. I'm on the Front Lines. I Have No Plan for This. The NewYorkTimes. https://www.nytimes.com/2020/03/24/opinion/coronavirus-hospital-visits.html?auth=login-email. Published March 24, 2020.

62. Columbia Journalism. "These Patients are Alone": A Doctor Talks About COVID-19 Diagnoses, Treatments, and Closed Doors. Medium. https://medium.com/columbiajourn/these-patients-are-alone-a-doctor-talks-about-covid-19-diagnoses-treatments-and-closed-doors-cb9589a72a99. Published April 17, 2020.

63. Contrera J. N95 masks save lives. So why are they still hard to get this far into a pandemic? The Washington Post. https://www.washingtonpost.com/graphics/2020/local/news/n-95-shortage-covid/. Published September 21, 2020.

64. Ariana Eunjung Cha MM. Hospital workers battling coronavirus turn to bandannas, sports goggles and homemade face shields amidshortages.TheWashingtonPost. https://www.washingtonpost.com/health/2020/03/19/hospital-workers-battling-coronavirus-turn-bandanas-sports-goggles-homemade-face-shields-amid-shortages/. Published March 20, 2020.

Chapter Ten
Strategies to Combat COVID-19

65. Simpson TF. Ventricular Arrhythmia Risk Due to Hydroxychloroquine-Azithromycin Treatment For COVID-19. American College of Cardiology. https://www.acc.org/latest-in-cardiology/articles/2020/03/27/14/00/ventricular-arrhythmia-risk-due-to-hydroxychloroquine-azithromycin-treatment-for-covid-19. Published March 29, 2020.

66. Kiley JP. NIH halts clinical trial of hydroxychloroquine. National Institutes of Health. https://www.nih.gov/news-events/news-releases/nih-halts-clinical-trial-hydroxychloroquine. Published June 20, 2020.

67. Bahrampour Juybari K, Pourhanifeh MH, Hosseinzadeh A, Hemati K, Mehrzadi S. Melatonin potentials against viral infections including COVID-19: Current evidence and new findings.Virusresearch. https://www.ncbi.nlm.nih.gov/pmc/articles/PMC7405774/. Published October 2, 2020.

68. Carr AC. A new clinical trial to test high-dose vitamin C in patients with COVID-19. Critical care (London, England). https://www.ncbi.nlm.nih.gov/pmc/articles/PMC7137406/. Published April 7, 2020.

69. Feyaerts AF, Luyten W. Vitamin C as prophylaxis and adjunctivemedicaltreatmentforCOVID-19?Nutrition. https://www.sciencedirect.com/science/article/pii/S0899900720 302318. Published July 25, 2020.

70. Velthuis AJWte, Sjoerd H. E. van den Worm, Sims AC, Baric RS, Snijder EJ, Hemert MJvan. Zn2+ Inhibits Coronavirus and Arterivirus RNA Polymerase Activity In Vitro and Zinc Ionophores Block the Replication of These Viruses in Cell

Culture. PLOS Pathogens. https://journals.plos.org/plospathogens/article?id=10.1371%2Fjournal.ppat.1001176. Published November 4, 2010.

71. staff SX. Scientists evaluate the perspectives of zinc intake for COVID-19 prevention. Medical Xpress - medical research advancesandhealthnews. https://medicalxpress.com/news/2020-07-scientists-perspectives-zinc-intake-covid-.html. Published July 14, 2020.

72. Skalny AV, Rink L, Ajsuvakova OP, et al. Zinc and respiratory tract infections: Perspectives for COVID-19 (Review). International Journal of Molecular Medicine. https://www.spandidos-publications.com/10.3892/ijmm.2020.4575. Published July 1, 2020.

73. Busko M. Low Vitamin D in COVID-19 Predicts ICU Admission, Poor Survival. Medscape. https://www.medscape.com/viewarticle/937567. Published September 17, 2020.

74. David O. Meltzer MD. Association of Vitamin D Status and Other Clinical Characteristics With COVID-19 Test Results. JAMA Network Open.

75. https://jamanetwork.com/journals/jamanetworkopen/fullarticle/2770157. Published September 3, 2020.

76. Cennimo DJ. What is the role of the IL-6 inhibitor tocilizumab (Actemra) in the treatment of coronavirus disease 2019 (COVID-19)? Latest Medical News, Clinical Trials, Guidelines -Todayon Medscape.https://www.medscape.com/answers/2500114-197457/what-is-the-role-of-the-il-6-inhibitor-tocilizumab-actemra-in-the-treatment-of-coronavirus-disease-2019-covid-19. Published October 18, 2020.

77. The RECOVERY Collaborative Group, Author AffiliationsFrom the Nuffield Department of Medicine (P.H.).

Dexamethasone in Hospitalized Patients with Covid-19 - Preliminary Report: NEJM. NewEnglandJournalofMedicine. https://www.nejm.org/doi/full/10.1056/NEJMoa2021436. Published July 17, 2020.

78. Rico-Mesa JS, Rosas D, Ahmadian-Tehrani A, White A, Anderson AS, Chilton R. The Role of Anticoagulation in COVID-19-Induced Hypercoagulability. Current cardiology reports. https://www.ncbi.nlm.nih.gov/pmc/articles/PMC7298694/. Published June 17, 2020.

79. Beigel JH, Al. E, for the ACTT-1 Study Group Members*, et al. Remdesivir for the Treatment of Covid-19 - Final Report: NEJM.NewEnglandJournalofMedicine. https://www.nejm.org/doi/full/10.1056/NEJMoa2007764. Published May 27, 2020.

80. Liu STH, Lin H-M, Baine I, et al. Convalescent plasma treatment of severe COVID-19: a propensity score–matched control study. Nature News. https://www.nature.com/articles/s41591-020-1088-9. Published September 15, 2020.

81. Center for Biologics Evaluation and Research. Investigational COVID-19 Convalescent Plasma - Emergency INDs. U.S. Food and Drug Administration. https://www.fda.gov/vaccines-blood-biologics/investigational-new-drug-ind-or-device-exemption-ide-process-cber/recommendations-investigational-covid-19-convalescent-plasma.

82. Damian Garde @damiangarde and Matthew Herper @matthewherper, Garde D, Herper M, et al. Large study suggests blood plasma can help treat Covid-19, with caveats. STAT. https://www.statnews.com/2020/08/13/large-study-suggests-convalescent-plasma-can-help-treat-covid-19-with-caveats/. Published August 13, 2020.

83. MichaelJ.Joyner,M.D.MayoClinic. https://www.mayo.edu/research/faculty/joyner-michael-j-m-d/bio-00078027. Published April 23, 2020.

84. https://www.who.int/docs/default-source/coronaviruse/situation-reports/20200306-sitrep-46-covid19.pdf?sfvrsn=96b04adf_4#:~:text=For%20COVID%2D19%2C,infections%2C%20requiring%20ventilation.

85. Brinkman C. Capturing a sneeze: Edgerton Center. Capturing a sneezeEdgertonCenter. https://edgerton.mit.edu/how_disease_epidemics_move_through_air. Published March 31, 2020.

86. Bourouiba L. Turbulent Gas Clouds and Respiratory Pathogen Emissions.JAMA. https://jamanetwork.com/journals/jama/fullarticle/2763852. Published May 12, 2020.

87. Ningthoujam R. COVID 19 can spread through breathing, talking, study estimates. Current medicine research and practice. https://www.ncbi.nlm.nih.gov/pmc/articles/PMC7205645/. Published 2020.

88. Zhou R, Li F, Chen F, et al. Viral dynamics in asymptomatic patients with COVID-19. International journal of infectious diseases : IJID : official publication of the International Society forInfectiousDiseases. https://www.ncbi.nlm.nih.gov/pmc/articles/PMC7211726/. Published July 2020.

89. COVID-19 Pandemic Planning Scenarios. Centers for Disease Control and Prevention. https://www.cdc.gov/coronavirus/2019-ncov/hcp/planning-scenarios.html.

90. Food Worker Handwashing in Restaurants. Centers for Disease ControlandPrevention. https://www.cdc.gov/nceh/ehs/ehsnet/plain_language/food-worker-handwashing-in-restaurants.html. Published August 26, 2020.

91. Show Me the Science. Centers for Disease Control and Prevention.
https://www.cdc.gov/handhygiene/science/index.html.
Published November 26, 2019.

92. Scientific Brief: SARS-CoV-2 and Potential Airborne Transmission. Centers for Disease Control and Prevention. https://www.cdc.gov/coronavirus/2019-ncov/more/scientific-brief-sars-cov-2.html.

93. Are outdoor gatherings safe? Here's what experts say. Advisory Board Daily Briefing. https://www.advisory.com/daily-briefing/2020/07/17/outdoor-gathering. Published July 16, 2020.

94. Stadnytskyi V, Bax CE, Bax A, Anfinrud P. The airborne lifetime of small speech droplets and their potential importance inSARS-CoV-2transmission.PNAS.
https://www.pnas.org/content/117/22/11875. Published June 2, 2020.

95. Nishiura H, Oshitani H, Kobayashi T, et al. Closed environments facilitate secondary transmission of coronavirus disease 2019 (COVID-19).medRxiv.
https://www.medrxiv.org/content/10.1101/2020.02.28.20029272v2. Published January 1, 2020.

96. Sheikh K. Talking Can Generate Coronavirus Droplets That Linger Up to 14 Minutes. The New York Times. https://www.nytimes.com/2020/05/14/health/coronavirus-infections.html. Published May 14, 2020.

97. Stay safe, have fun during the COVID-19 pandemic. Mayo Clinic.https://www.mayoclinic.org/diseases-conditions/coronavirus/in-depth/safe-activities-during-covid19/art-20489385. Published August 5, 2020.

98. Social Distancing, Quarantine, and Isolation. Centers for Disease Control and Prevention. https://www.cdc.gov/coronavirus/2019-

ncov/prevent-getting-sick/social-distancing.html. Published July 15, 2020.

99. Qureshi Z, Bourouiba L, Greenhalgh T, Larwood JPJ, Temple R, Jones N. What is the evidence to support the 2-metre social distancing rule to reduce COVID-19 transmission? CEBM. https://www.cebm.net/covid-19/what-is-the-evidence-to-support-the-2-metre-social-distancing-rule-to-reduce-covid-19-transmission/. Published June 25, 2020.

100. Hogan A. How much of the coronavirus does it take to make you sick? STAT. https://www.statnews.com/2020/04/14/how-much-of-the-coronavirus-does-it-take-to-make-you-sick/. Published April 13, 2020.

101. Schröder I. COVID-19: A Risk Assessment Perspective. JournalofChemicalHealth&Safety. https://www.ncbi.nlm.nih.gov/pmc/articles/PMC7216769/. Published May 11, 2020.

102. Sanche S, Lin YT, Xu C, Romero-Severson E, Hengartner N, Ke R. High Contagiousness and Rapid Spread of Severe Acute Respiratory Syndrome Coronavirus 2. Emerging infectious diseases. https://www.ncbi.nlm.nih.gov/pmc/articles/PMC7323562/. Published July 2020.

103. Liu Y, Gayle AA, Wilder-Smith A, Rocklöv J. reproductive number of COVID-19 is higher compared to SARS coronavirus. OUPAcademic. https://academic.oup.com/jtm/article/27/2/taaa021/5735319. Published February 13, 2020.

104. Wang J, Pan L, Tang S, Ji JS, Shi X. Mask use during COVID-19: A risk adjusted strategy. Environmental pollution (Barking,Essex:1987). https://www.ncbi.nlm.nih.gov/pmc/articles/PMC7314683/. Published November 2020.

Directly Observed Self-isolation and Contact-Tracing (DOS-CT)

105. Department of Health. Directly Observed Therapy (DOT): InformationforHealthCareProviders. https://www.health.ny.gov/publications/3705/. https://www.health.ny.gov/publications/3705.pdf.

106. The top 10 causes of death. World Health Organization. https://www.who.int/news-room/fact-sheets/detail/the-top-10-causes-of-death. Published May 24, 2018.

107. Tuberculosis mortality nearly halved since 1990. World Health Organization. https://www.who.int/news-room/detail/28-10-2015-tuberculosis-mortality-nearly-halved-since-1990. Published October 28, 2015.

108. TB Incidence in the U.S. Centers for Disease Control and Prevention.https://www.cdc.gov/tb/statistics/tbcases.htm. Published September 6, 2019.

109. Chaulk CP, Moore-Rice K, Rizzo R, Chaisson R. Eleven years of community-based directly observed therapy for tuberculosis.JAMA. https://pubmed.ncbi.nlm.nih.gov/7674524/. Published 1995.

110. Loddenkemper R, Sagebiel D, Brendel A. Strategies against multidrug-resistant tuberculosis. European Respiratory Society. https://erj.ersjournals.com/content/20/36_suppl/66s. Published July 1, 2002.

111. Sterling TR. Drug-Resistant Tuberculosis in New York City:LessonstoRemember.OUPAcademic. https://academic.oup.com/cid/article/42/12/1711/294685. Published June 15, 2006.

112. Burman WJ;Dalton CB;Cohn DL;Butler JR;Reves RR; A cost-effectiveness analysis of directly observed therapy vs self-

administered therapy for treatment of tuberculosis. Chest. https://pubmed.ncbi.nlm.nih.gov/9228359/.

113. Frieden TR, Hamburg MA, Washko RM, Fujiwara PI. Tuberculosis in New York City--turning the tide. The New Englandjournalofmedicine. https://pubmed.ncbi.nlm.nih.gov/7791840/. Published July 27, 1995.

114. Guo X;Yang Y;Takiff HE;Zhu M;Ma J;Zhong T;Fan Y;Wang J;Liu S; A Comprehensive App That Improves Tuberculosis Treatment Management Through Video-Observed Therapy: Usability Study. JMIR mHealth and uHealth. https://pubmed.ncbi.nlm.nih.gov/32735222/.

115. Electronic Directly Observed Therapy for Active TB Disease. Centers for Disease Control and Prevention. https://www.cdc.gov/nchhstp/highimpactprevention/promising-hip-intervention.html. Published October 4, 2019.

116. Moore RD, Chaulk CP, Griffiths R, Cavalcante S, R CE. American Journal of Respiratory and Critical Care Medicine. American journal of respiratory and critical care medicine. https://www.atsjournals.org/doi/abs/10.1164/ajrccm.154.4.8887600.

117. Gasner MR;Maw KL;Feldman GE;Fujiwara PI;Frieden TR; The use of legal action in New York City to ensure treatment of tuberculosis. The New England journal of medicine. https://pubmed.ncbi.nlm.nih.gov/9929527/. Published February 4, 1999.

118. Danmeng M, Ning D, Huixia S. In Depth: How Shanghai showed China how to deal with coronavirus. Nikkei Asia. https://asia.nikkei.com/Spotlight/Caixin/In-Depth-How-Shanghai-showed-China-how-to-deal-with-coronavirus. Published March 21, 2020.

119. Shen Y, Additional informationFundingThis work was supported by Shanghai Science and Technology Committee

under Grant 20431900403, References. Epidemiology and clinical course of COVID-19 in Shanghai, China. Taylor & Francis. https://www.tandfonline.com/doi/full/10.1080/22221751.2020.1787103. Published June 23, 2020.

Chapter Eleven

Let us Fix It – It is About Time!

120. Rosenthal BM. This Hospital Cost $52 Million. It Treated 79VirusPatients.TheNewYorkTimes. https://www.nytimes.com/2020/07/21/nyregion/coronavirus-hospital-usta-queens.html. Published July 21, 2020.

121. Ellison A. $52M field hospital in New York treated only 79 COVID-19 patients: A temporary hospital that opened in April to treat COVID-19 patients in New York City treated only 79 patients during the month it was open, according to The New YorkTimes. Becker'sHospitalReview. https://www.beckershospitalreview.com/patient-flow/52m-field-hospital-in-new-york-treated-only-79-covid-19-patients.html. Published July 21, 2020.

122. Michael R. Sisak TAP. Many field hospitals went largely unused, will be shut down. Military Times.

123. https://www.militarytimes.com/news/coronavirus/2020/04/29/many-field-hospitals-went-largely-unused-will-be-shut-down/. Published April 29, 2020.

124. 1918 Pandemic Influenza: Three Waves. Centers for DiseaseControlandPrevention. https://www.cdc.gov/flu/pandemic-resources/1918-commemoration/three-waves.htm. Published May 11, 2018.

125. www.cdc.gov/flu/pandemic-resources/1918-commemoration/images/death-chart.jpg.

126. Shockandawe.Wikipedia. https://en.wikipedia.org/wiki/Shock_and_awe. Published October 8, 2020.

Chapter Twelve

The Warriors, The Martyrs – All Heroes

127. McNamara A. The CDC says over 600 health care workers have died from the coronavirus. This doctor has counted hundreds more. CBS News. https://www.cbsnews.com/news/dr-claire-rezba-tracks-healthcare-workers-coronavirus-deaths/. Published August 14, 2020.

128. CDC COVID Data Tracker. Centers for Disease Control and Prevention.https://covid.cdc.gov/covid-data-tracker/?CDC_AA_refVal=https%3A%2F%2Fwww.cdc.gov%2Fcoronavirus%2F2019-ncov%2Fcases-updates%2Fcases-in-us.html. Published October 18, 2020.

Epilogue

129. La Monica PR. Vaccine maker backed by Bill & Melinda Gatessoars40%.CNN. https://www.cnn.com/2020/08/17/investing/curevac-vaccine-stock/index.html. Published August 17, 2020.

130. The case for physician CEOs: In today's healthcare climate, who is best suited to lead? Becker's Hospital Review. https://www.beckershospitalreview.com/hospital-management-administration/the-case-for-physician-ceos.html.

131. Goodall AH. Physician-Leaders and Hospital Performance: Is There an Association. http://ftp.iza.org/dp5830.pdf.

132. National Health Expenditures 2018 Highlights. cms.gov. https://www.cms.gov/files/document/highlights.pdf.

133. Frakt A. The Astonishingly High Administrative Costs of U.S. Health Care. The New York Times. https://www.nytimes.com/2018/07/16/upshot/costs-health-care-us.html. Published July 16, 2018.

134. Defense Budget Overview. dod.defense.gov. https://dod.defense.gov/Portals/1/Documents/pubs/FY2019-Budget-Request-Overview-Book.pdf.

135. Sull D, Homkes R, Sull C. Why Strategy Execution Unravels-and What to Do About It. Harvard Business Review. https://hbr.org/2015/03/why-strategy-execution-unravelsand-what-to-do-about-it?cm_sp=Nav+Landing-_-Links-_-Featured+Item. Published September 7, 2017.